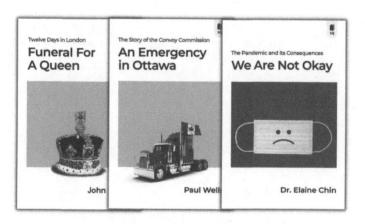

WE ARE NOT
OKAY

WE ARE NOT
OKAY

The Pandemic and its Consequences

DR. ELAINE CHIN

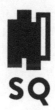

SQ

sh.
SUTHERLAND HOUSE

Sutherland House
416 Moore Ave., Suite 205
Toronto, ON M4G 1C9

First edition, June 2023

If you are interested in inviting one of our authors to a live event or media appearance, please contact sranasinghe@sutherlandhousebooks.com and visit our website at sutherlandhousebooks.com for more information about our authors and their schedules.

We acknowledge the support of the Government of Canada.

Manufactured in Canada
Cover designed by Lena Yang
Book composed by Karl Hunt

ISBN 978-1-990823-36-7
eBook 978-1-990823-46-6

ABOUT THE AUTHOR

Dr. Elaine Chin is a one of North America's leading medical experts and respected thought leaders in the space of personalized medicine. She is the author of the *Globe & Mail* Top 10 bestseller *Lifelines: Unlocking the Secret of Your Telomeres for a Longer, Healthier Life* and a wellness expert on Bell Media's *CP24 Toronto* and *CTV Your Morning*.

Also by Dr. Elaine Chin

*Lifelines: Unlocking the Secret of Your Telomeres
for a Longer, Healthier Life*

*Welcome Back!: How to Reboot Your Physical and
Mental Well-Being for a Post-Pandemic World*

This book is dedicated to my amazing publisher and editor, Kenneth Whyte. He believed in my knowledge and encouraged me to improve my writing. Thanks to him, I'm a better communicator today. This marks my third book, one he claims will make me a legitimate author, finally! Thank you, Ken, for being my mentor and friend.

CONTENTS

CONTENTS

INTRODUCTION

It has been more than three years since the World Health Organization (WHO) declared the COVID-19 pandemic and we're still not sure how it began. The initial theory was that it originated in a zoonotic (animal to human) spillover from bats and spread through the Wuhan wet market, where such animals are prepared and served. Almost as soon as that theory gained traction, there were suspicions that it was false or, at least, not the whole story. The leading alternative theory has been that the virus emerged from a lab leak at the Wuhan Institute of Virology, which studies and experiments on specimens of coronavirus in bats.

Through most of the pandemic, mainstream scientists and science organizations viewed the lab leak origin as a conspiracy theory, but evidence for it is building. In February 2023, the *Wall Street Journal* reported on a classified document from the US Department of Energy that said a lab leak is the most likely explanation for the virus' origin and initial spread.[1] The department qualified its assessment by saying that its conclusion was reached with "low confidence."[2]

Critics of the department's report and the lab leak theory note that other branches of the US government still favour natural transmission as the most likely origin of the virus or are noncommittal on the question of where it came from. Some observers have called the report racist for pinning the worldwide pandemic on the Chinese government and accusing it of a massive cover-up.

In my view, there is nothing crazy about the lab leak theory. The Chinese government is incredibly secretive and controlling and it is not hard to imagine that it would have moved quickly to avoid embarrassment by obscuring COVID's origins and suggesting an alternate theory.

Reasonable people might disagree. The point is that the origins of the virus are still under debate.

The controversy has fed into distrust of the Chinese government, the World Health Organization, and even our own public health authorities. There have been allegations of a cover-up. A lot of people noticed that the lab leak theory was suppressed during the first half of the pandemic and that anyone who promoted it was dismissed as a crank. That approach, admits former WHO advisor Jamie Metzl, was a significant tactical mistake which created a "huge problem" in communications and credibility.[3]

The problem is ongoing. China continues to stonewall, leaving scientists with insufficient evidence to draw conclusions. The journal *Nature* reported in February 2023 that the WHO had "quietly shelved" its plans to continue its investigation into the origins of what is formally known as SARS-CoV2. WHO denied the report and in March urged the Chinese government to release all relevant information on the origins of the pandemic.[4] Meanwhile, a new theory has emerged that has nothing to do with either bats or lab leaks: there is compelling evidence that raccoon dogs, also available in Wuhan's live animal market, may have been responsible for the zoonotic transmission.[5]

People whose lives were altered by what transpired in the time of COVID-19 and especially the families of the millions who died deserve to know the truth about its origins. I have "low confidence" that we will ever get it. That the source of virus remains unknown and a subject of bitter controversy three years after its emergence is, unfortunately, typical of the entire pandemic experience.

We're still counting how many people got sick and how many died as a result of contracting the virus. We are still learning about the after-effects of COVID-19 infection; not only Long COVID but damage to lungs, hearts, kidneys, brains, and skin, as well as increased risk of diabetes and weakened immune systems. We are still measuring the massive impact of delayed patient care and conditions left undiagnosed as a result of the lockdowns and the medical resources diverted to fighting COVID-19. We are still assessing the consequences to health-care workers, our health-care system, our long-term care homes and their staffs.

The social and mental health repercussions of COVID-19 are often harder to measure than the medical phenomena, but they are nonetheless real. People have been grief-stricken, traumatized, angry, enraged, and miserable. Years of social isolation have had disturbing effects, especially on the young and the elderly. A whole range of mental health markers, from anxiety to suicide ideation, trended the wrong way. Substance abuse and violent crimes spiked. It has all left people wary of one another and our institutions, whether government, health authorities, or the media. The whole of our public sphere remains feverish and quarrelsome.

And then there are the economic consequences. A global recession. Declines in economic output. Supply chain disruptions. A bear market. Inflation. Businesses closed or crippled. Jobs lost. Bank accounts drained. The disappearance and only partial re-appearance of the common workplace. It has been one blow after another in a short time.

The pandemic has been an ordeal unlike any in our lifetimes. Every person, family, and nation on earth has been traumatized by COVID-19, although its effects are often invisible. Not one individual has been spared. This book examines how the pandemic has left us beaten, broken, scarred, and sick. Admitting that we are not okay and taking a true inventory of the consequences of the pandemic are the first steps toward getting back to normal and preparing for the next one. Because there will undoubtedly be a next one.

CHAPTER ONE

WHAT HAPPENED

It would be nice if we could dismiss the impact of the pandemic by uttering thoughts and prayers for the sick and the dead and simply moving on as though it never happened. Many are trying to do just that. We've all become sick of COVID-19, literally or figuratively, and it's understandable that some would wish to never hear or speak of it again. But that is impossible.

Far too many people died and far too much damage was done. We owe it to the dead to never forget the pandemic. We also owe it to ourselves. After an event as serious as this, the best thing we can do is to fully understand the toll it took on us. If we are going to recover from the pandemic, regain our physical and mental health, and gather the strength to move ahead, we need to acknowledge that the last three years have been exceptional and hellishly difficult.

Let's review how we got here. What follows in this chapter is a slightly Ontario-centric account of the pandemic in Canada. This is not intended to slight my fellow citizens in other parts of the country or elsewhere in the world. It's a simple reflection of the fact that I live and work in Ontario and am most familiar with events here. It should be noted that while some parts of the country were hit harder than others and responses differed among provincial governments and populations, the successive waves of COVID-19 and the repeating pattern of lockdowns and loosened restrictions occurred almost everywhere.

For most of us, the first inkling that a significant viral infection was on the loose in the world came from news stories in January 2020. The infection appeared to mimic other viruses that had come before. The

Chinese government seemed worried, although it was only reporting a few pneumonia cases.[1] The World Health Organization, too, attributed the illnesses to a mysterious form of pneumonia. It was an interesting story and maybe even concerning, but there were no alarm bells going off. The last respiratory virus pandemic had been the swine flu (H1N1) in 2009. While it had infected many people, we'd managed to bring it quickly under control and it had a relatively low death rate. Like the SARS virus pandemic (SARS-CoV1) of 2003, H1N1 hit hard and briefly in Asia and Canada and then disappeared. At the start of 2020, I was cautiously optimistic that history was on our side and all would turn out well.

We now know that the virus was already out of control in January 2020. Recent evidence has shown that it had been spreading through Europe months earlier. Retrospective testing of blood and respiratory samples indicates the virus was likely in Italy in September 2019 and in France by December.[2, 3]

On January 11, China reported the first death from the novel coronavirus. Nine days later, the Chinese government announced its finding that the virus could be spread directly from person to person. On January 21, the US confirmed its first case and on January 23, China imposed a strict lockdown in Wuhan and began construction of two new hospitals. A "Public Health Emergency of International Concern" was declared by the World Health Organization on January 30, 2020.[4]

Canada was immune to none of this. A fifty-six-year-old Toronto man who had recently traveled to Wuhan was confirmed as our first case on January 25.[5] He was admitted to Sunnybrook Hospital and placed in isolation. His wife became Canada's second case, a harbinger of eventual community spread. From my experience with the SARS outbreak in 2003, I had an inkling of how things would unfold. I sent a bulletin to my patients on January 26, warning of a potential "exponential curve" caused by community spread and advising against travel, and recommending the use of face masks. More travel cases were discovered in the days following,[6] including, on January 28, a British Columbia man in his forties.

Here, as elsewhere in the world, people were slow to take the virus seriously. The idea of a "wave" of COVID-19 had not yet penetrated the general consciousness. It would be almost two months from the first case to the first lockdown. The horrors of the pandemic would register gradually, ratcheting up tension and anxiety along the way.

The infamous Diamond Princess cruise ship was quarantined in Japan during the first week in February. In the second week, the novel coronavirus was renamed COVID-19. The first US case of local transmission was confirmed on February 26, three days before the first American death was reported.

Canadians watched as more and more travel cases were reported, mostly from the United States.[7] We saw governments around the world begin to institute travel restrictions and bans and introduce isolation policies in a largely futile effort to halt community spread. On February 27, I sent another note to my patients advising that we had a genuine pandemic on our hands: "While professional agencies around the world have not yet called it a pandemic (which has huge economic implications), academically and practically, we are there."

Wave One

March 11 was a watershed. The WHO upgraded COVID-19 from an emergency of international concern to a global pandemic and infectious disease expert Dr. Anthony Fauci told the United States Congress that there were already 647 confirmed cases in the US and that the outbreak was about to get much worse. As if to prove Fauci's point, the NBA cancelled a game that evening between the Oklahoma Thunder and the Utah Jazz because one player, Rudy Gobert, had tested positive. Hours later, the NBA suspended its entire season. From there, things got really bad, really fast.

Cancellations and shutdowns were announced everywhere. President Donald Trump declared a national emergency on March 13, forty-eight hours before the Centers for Disease Control and Prevention warned against large gatherings. Through the middle of March, new phrases like "shelter in place" joined our vocabulary. Italy's death toll went through the roof, Manhattan emerged as the epicentre of the US outbreak and Japan postponed its Olympic games.

On March 13, two days after the WHO had made the pandemic official, our federal government, acting on the advice of the Public Health

Agency of Canada (PHAC) recommended that Canadians abstain from non-essential travel. On March 16, it recommended fourteen days of self-isolation for travelers entering Canada. Two days more and the border was shut down to all except Americans and the first financial supports for individuals and businesses affected by the pandemic were announced.[8]

That the seriousness of the virus dawned on us only gradually did not make it any less shocking when its scope became evident. The tenor of news reports and our own thoughts darkened as the case counts grew. COVID-19 was no longer some remote, foreign menace, but a clear and present danger that was beginning to fill our hospitals. Canada's first COVID-19 death was an elderly man in a Vancouver nursing home, portending carnage for our most vulnerable population. "Not a cause for panic," read the CBC headline, perhaps optimistically.[9]

On March 17, Ontario and Alberta declared states of emergency, the first provinces in Canada to do so. Lockdowns had begun at least two weeks too late. They were expected to be brief. We were inundated with messaging like "two weeks to stop the spread" and told to wash our hands frequently. Masks were not yet emphasized by public health authorities.

There was a sudden rush to stock up on basic household supplies. Toilet paper, in particular, was highly coveted. The spectacle of empty grocery shelves, something never before seen in most people's lives, heightened the alarm and led to hoarding, exacerbating the emerging supply chain problems. People concerned about shopping "in person" were frustrated by the challenges of finding alternatives, given how underdeveloped and overstretched our shopping and delivery services were in that moment. People most in need of those services—seniors and individuals in quarantine—were often unable to access them.

By April 2, global cases hit one million and obscure institutional websites such as the Johns Hopkins Coronavirus Resource Center became the hottest destinations on the Internet. Notwithstanding the fear and anxiety of those early weeks—the hauntingly empty streets and stores and offices, the new paths on lawns and boulevards where people were veering off the pavement to stay six feet from their fellow pedestrians—there was also the exhilaration of a fully shared experience. We were all in it together. People came out of their front doors and onto their balconies in the evening to bang pots and pans and cheer health-care workers. Initial panic over loss of income for those who were unable to work due to lockdowns eased as the federal government passed its first COVID-19 aid bill, pledging an initial $107 billion in support.[10] Public health authorities such as the federal Chief Public Health Officer Dr. Theresa Tam became national celebrities.

The initial advice we were given on how best to prevent infection was unhelpful. Non-medical mask usage was discouraged, supposedly because they were ineffective and provided a false sense of security. Early guidance from the World Health Organization was that COVID-19 was transmitted primarily through "respiratory droplets" and human contact, especially coughs and sneezes, and that it didn't linger in the air. Following that reasoning, our government officials assured the public that keeping six feet apart would do the trick. Masks were described as "optional."

The WHO's guidance was pointedly challenged by some experts in viral transmission, including Dr. Donald Milton, an infectious disease aerobiologist at the University of Maryland's School of Public Health. "I think they are talking out of their hats," he said.[11] Milton and others argued that there was reason to believe the virus was airborne—that it was capable of floating in the air for minutes, if not hours at a time.

Nobody got everything right in the pandemic but I tended to agree with the dissenters to the WHO guidance, again because of my experience with SARS in 2003 and also because a patient asked me to help her manage a COVID-19 outbreak in the call centre she ran. This facility housed around a thousand people but now had only about a quarter of its staff on-site to operate essential services, including suicide hotlines and financial services. Within days, we went from two or three cases to eight. The facility voluntarily closed for cleaning, but soon public health authorities requested an extended closure. The final case count reached thirty-two before the call center was reopened two weeks later.

This may not seem like a remarkable COVID story, but what struck me, and was not discussed by health officials at the time, was the information we gathered on how the infection scattered across the floor plan of a 40,000-square-foot facility. The workers were socially distanced in an indoor setting and yet those who tested positive worked in different locations all over the building, evidence for the virus's airborne nature.

In any event, it was not until April 7, several weeks after lockdowns began and nearly two and a half months since the first Canadian case, that PHAC and Dr. Tam finally recommended the use of non-medical masks. Even then, the recommendation was couched in weak language with the proviso that mask use was still only in addition to primary prevention measures like handwashing.[12] We were washing our hands fifty times a day. We were washing everything, including our groceries. Hand sanitizer was sold out everywhere.

It would be several months more before health authorities indirectly acknowledged that social distancing and constant washing of hands and use of hand sanitizer were not adequate to control the spread of the disease. Everyone now needed to wear masks, especially indoors. High-efficiency particulate air (HEPA) filters needed to be installed in indoor workplaces, schools, and homes.

This was the first of many times I suspected public health agencies around the world, including in Canada, were holding back lifesaving information by around two to four weeks. I believe, as some news outlets reported, that they were trying to manage or stagger the release of important scientific information in the hopes of preventing panic.[13] If so, it was a mistake at such an unprecedented time in our lives. Public health officials had no right to control the narrative in this way and their attempts to do so later resulted in a catastrophic loss of trust, particularly among physicians and health-care workers on the front lines.

In retrospect, it appears that the guidance of public health agencies on masks in the early stages of the pandemic was influenced at least in part by the availability of personal protective equipment (PPE). We held off telling people to wear masks simply because there were not enough of them for everyone in the country, let alone the world. No one had stockpiled masks for a rainy day and our just-in-time inventory model doesn't work during a global pandemic.

Even with health authorities calling masks optional, there was high demand for them, especially at hospitals and nursing homes. Many doctors were trying to lay in supplies. In maybe the most bizarre episode of the pandemic for me, I found myself trying to import a few skids of medical-grade masks in March 2020.

Naively, I thought getting a few cartons of masks wouldn't be a problem. I simply contacted a friendly medical supplier who managed to quickly secure an order for five million masks. It seemed straightforward: arrange a line of credit, put down a deposit, and the shipment would come in a few weeks. I thought I'd get what I needed and help Ottawa and the provincial governments in Ontario and British Columbia with their supplies. I wondered aloud why the Canadian government was having so much trouble procuring PPE, returning from China many times with either fake or damaged PPE, and once even an empty cargo plane. I was about to learn a lesson in global trade as practiced in a pandemic.

We had our bulk order on the tarmac at the airport in Shanghai, ready to be shipped. Suddenly our five million masks disappeared. It turned out we were outbid. A surprise cash offer four times our agreed upon price short-circuited our deal. Somebody pulled up with a truck and loaded our pallets for delivery on another plane. It was the craziest thing. To this day, we have no idea where the masks wound up.

By mid-April, it was clear that the initial "two weeks" lockdown messaging was a sham and that we were going to be stuck in isolation for the foreseeable future. The economic consequences were profound. About 3.1 million Canadians either lost their jobs or had their hours reduced in the first months of the pandemic. The value of firms trading on the TSX fell 37 percent in a month. A survey by the Canadian Federation of Independent Businesses indicated that 70 percent of small businesses lost at least 30 percent of their revenues. Women and minority populations were especially hard hit. Alcohol sales jumped 17.5 percent.[14]

Childcare soon became an issue. Health-care workers and essential workers with children were especially challenged.[15] Schools were shut down on extremely short notice and additional assistance did not come quickly enough. Even those working from home found it a challenge to balance work and family life. Children appearing on work Zoom calls became a common and, thankfully, accepted sight.

As spring approached, we became more accustomed to new COVID-19 routines. Day-to-day survival became a game of staving off boredom or managing the new reality of working and/or schooling from home. Meal kit delivery services became incredibly popular. People ordered takeout to support local restaurants in danger of going under with their doors closed, or learned to appreciate the novel experience of streetside outdoor dining. Baking bread and making cocktails were two of the top new hobbies, giving us something to occupy our minds and fill our stomachs. Like toilet paper before them, flour and yeast suddenly disappeared from grocery store aisles as people baked and ate, often to the detriment of their waistlines. [16]

Difficult as these adjustments to daily living were to working families, the vast majority of people managed to cope reasonably well. It was a different story in the nation's over-crowded emergency rooms and ICUs, where ventilators were in short supply and front-line health-care workers were struggling to keep up with the flood of patients. The lockdowns were extended, largely to "flatten the curve" of new cases and to ensure critical care was available to those who needed it.

The worst of the first wave was felt in our nursing homes. On May 7, the *Toronto Star* reported that 4,167 Canadians had thus far died of COVID-19, with 82 percent of the victims in long-term care settings, the worst performance among the fourteen countries surveyed.[17] Our nursing homes were the abattoirs of the first wave, a shameful legacy that we have not reconciled to this day.

Just as shocking as the number of deaths in long-term care facilities were the deplorable conditions suffered by residents. Many facilities couldn't keep staff and those workers who remained on the job were overstretched and burnt out. The Canadian Armed Forces were called to floundering long-term care homes in Ontario and Quebec. What they encountered, as reported on May 26, was shocking. Our most vulnerable populations were subjected to horrific conditions. "Patients [were] observed crying for help with staff not responding for 30 mins to over two hours."[18] Basic hygiene had been neglected: some residents were left sitting in soiled diapers; some had not been bathed for weeks or had untreated bed sores attributable to prolonged bed rest; still others were malnourished. Cockroaches and rotten food were found in the facilities. Some residents with COVID-19 were allowed to wander the hallways. Employees were re-using personal protective equipment, and moving from unit to unit with contaminated gear.[19] "Degrading or inappropriate comments" were directed at residents. There were accounts of "forceful feeding," resulting in "audible choking."

Even in the context of a once-in-a-century pandemic, these reports of abuse, neglect, and bullying were appalling. [20]

The elderly were society's lost members in these months. Those who caught COVID-19 often died alone in hospital, unable to receive visits from family or friends. Even those fortunate enough to dodge the virus and live in better-run facilities were virtual inmates, shut in their rooms with no company beyond their televisions. The first signs of a breakdown in public spirit appeared that spring as families despaired for the welfare of the elderly. Canada recorded 8,839 deaths during the first wave, the vast majority of them among residents of care homes. [21]

(For a time, it appeared there would be a silver living—that the shocking reports of tragedies in our long-term care homes would stick in our minds and lead to real change. This was not to be. The *Globe & Mail* reported early in 2023 that while the federal government unveiled new national standards for long-term care aimed at addressing systemic problems exposed by the coronavirus pandemic, there is no plan to make the standards mandatory. [22])

Some of us were affected directly by these incidents and deaths, but for the vast majority of Canadians, they remained distant, almost abstract. The first wave hit its peak on May 30, 2020, after which the daily count of new cases started a gradual decline. The NBA and NHL announced plans to continue competition safely in bubbles. We started to feel slightly normal again and the warm weather brought more people outside.

On May 23, 2020, thousands packed Toronto's Trinity Bellwoods Park. It was a beautiful day, and, clearly, Torontonians were desperate for a taste of normalcy. We know in retrospect that being outdoors on a sunny day was a very safe activity, but there was a lot of confusion then about what constituted safe activity and what didn't. The *Toronto Sun* splashed the Trinity Bellwoods gathering on its front page. [23] The image of masses of people congregating in relatively close quarters was triggering for many, creating fears of a new outbreak. It was a sign of conflict to come. [24]

Lockdowns started to lift in June in British Columbia and July in Ontario. The summer felt almost normal. Many small businesses were cautiously optimistic that with online and curbside shopping, outdoor dining, and federal support for wages and rent, they would be able to survive and move on. We didn't fully appreciate yet that the first wave, relatively speaking, was the calm before the storm.

Physicians and health authorities warned that there would likely be a new wave of infections later in the year. I wrote to my patients: "I guarantee you we are in no way out of this pandemic and the risk of you succumbing to COVID-19 remains present, but for now, it's just hidden."

Wave Two

The first of many strains or "variants" of COVID-19 would be named with the Greek alphabet rather than numerical designations. Alpha (B.1.1.7) joined us for the winter of 2020-21.[25] It took four months in the middle of 2020 for Canada's total case count to rise from 100,000 to 200,000 in mid-October. By mid-November, in less than four weeks, we had jumped to 300,000 cases. On November 27, Ontario reported a record-breaking daily case count of 1,855 new infections.[26] True, we were testing more at this point, but the rate of hospitalizations made the reality of this new wave clear. In early December, Ontario's ICU occupancy hit 203, well above the regular threshold of 150, at which point the province's health system is considered at capacity.[27]

We all knew, deep down, that another lockdown was inevitable. As I wrote to my patients, "You've seen this movie once already." Without vaccines and with cases, hospitalizations, and deaths exploding, Ontario, BC, and Quebec began imposing new restrictions in November. Thankfully, the first vaccines arrived much earlier than anyone expected—the greatest Christmas present we could have received.

On November 20, 2020, Pfizer-BioNTech applied to the US Food and Drug Administration for Emergency Use Authorization for its newly developed mRNA vaccine. This seemed miraculous at the time, as, until then, no vaccine had ever been produced so quickly.[28] The Pfizer product was the fruit of Operation Warp Speed, a US government program to expedite the development of COVID-19 vaccines. Warp Speed was perhaps the signature achievement of the Trump administration, which would otherwise prove to be a disaster on the COVID-19 file.

On December 9, 2020, Health Canada authorized the first COVID-19 vaccine in Canada.[29] The Pfizer-BioNTech vaccine was first administered to people in Quebec and Ontario starting on December 14, 2020, but most Canadians weren't able to access their first doses for several more months. In the meantime, our largest provinces had moved from increasing restrictions to full lockdowns, with prohibitions on in-person dining and closure of non-essential businesses. B.C. closed again in November. Ontario's new lockdown was declared on December 26, 2020, and initially scheduled to last for twenty-eight days. It was later extended for several weeks in some regions. We needed to buy time and manage the case load until we could acquire and distribute vaccines for all Canadians.

Like many front-line health personnel around the world, I noticed around this time that I was suffering certain effects from living and working with COVID-19. I wrote to my patients in January 2021 that, in retrospect, "I experienced some PTSD in the early months of this pandemic." I was recalling the fears of dying during SARS. "I wish it was otherwise," I wrote, "but I'm afraid I don't have good news to share. I fear 2021 will be worse, from an infection perspective. The more contagious strain appears to be taking hold."

The first months of 2021 were frantic. Case counts got so bad in Ontario that the province issued a stay-at-home order on January 14, 2021.[30] As many in the medical community had warned during the first wave, the second wave of COVID-19 exposed the fragility of our health system. ICUs overflowed and hospitalizations soared. Some hospitals were forced to cancel elective surgeries and procedures—anything deemed non-essential was cancelled or postponed to free resources for COVID-19 patients. The demand for testing exceeded our ability to deliver. Contact tracing became almost impossible due to the sheer numbers of people impacted. Health workers were facing burnout en masse. Some provinces implemented programs to provide mental health support for front-line personnel. We will discuss the impact of the pandemic on our health-care system in a later section of this book.

The we're-all-in-this-together vibe of the first wave did not survive the second. Cracks in society were evident. People were taking sides and the pandemic was now threatening to break us apart. In February 2021, Trinity Bible Chapel in Waterloo, Ontario, was hit with significant fines for holding services despite the limit on indoor gatherings. More of the same was happening in Alberta and three churches in B.C.'s Fraser valley were fined as well.[31]

To the extent there was good news, it was that residents and staff at long-term-care centres were receiving their first doses of vaccines. Ontario had jabbed all long-term-care residents and staff in the Greater Toronto Area by the end of January. This would go a long way toward stemming the horrific tide of death in those facilities.

Quebec began to open up again in February after the number of cases began to subside. Ontario's second lockdown was phased out by March 8. Wave two ended with a total of 13,312 deaths nationwide, nearly double the body count of the first wave. The true toll of the pandemic was becoming clear. More and more people had either been sick themselves or had lost someone to infection. At the end of this wave, we knew there were more variants on the horizon and that we were still a long way from getting out of this, but the vaccines were reason for hope.

Wave Three

Along with vaccines, new variants began to arrive. The Beta variant, first detected in South Africa, was carried to Canada in January 2021 by a person who had been visiting that country. Weeks later came Gamma, courtesy of a person who had been traveling in Brazil. The Delta variant arrived in British Columbia around April 1, 2021,[32] bringing with it heightened anxieties. We had been developing the vaccines quickly, but the virus was fighting back in its own way, mutating to avoid killing its hosts while increasing its infectiousness to survive. Delta had enhanced transmissibility, estimated at 40-60 percent above the Alpha variant.[33]

The Ontario COVID-19 Science Advisory Table noted a sharp uptick in Delta cases and announced on March 16, 2021, that a third wave was in progress.[34] Three weeks later, a third provincewide stay-at-home order was announced in Ontario. The repetitive nature of waves and the seesawing between lockdowns and openings was getting very old by now. Intolerance for all things COVID-19 had set in. There was frustration with conflicting advice from public health authorities, particularly over the use of masks, which were now mandatory in many circumstances, but also with regard to social interactions, quarantine measures, and travel restrictions. There was confusion over the precise meaning of phrases such as "flatten the curve" and "herd immunity" and their relation to the ongoing lockdowns.

The vaccines themselves were becoming politicized, especially once the skeptical realized that being vaxxed was going to be a de facto license to participate in society. As 2021 wore on, this became a full-on culture war. Former President Trump himself was booed at one of his own rallies when he mentioned that he had received vaccine doses.[35] These sentiments were supercharged in the United States but also spilled over into significant portions of Canadian society.

The vaccines were godsends, but not without problems. The Oxford Astra-Zeneca (AZ) viral vector vaccine arrived in Canada about one month before the new stay-at-home order, with the first doses being distributed to pharmacies in early March as part of a pilot program. The relatively slow rollout of mRNA vaccines meant that AZ doses, which were easier to store and available in greater numbers, became the first dose available to many Canadians. While it was better than nothing, the AZ vaccine was extremely controversial and legitimately concerning. In late 2020, South Africa had been swiped by the Beta strain. The AZ vaccine was ineffective against Beta and South Africa stopped using it.[36] Scientific logic would indicate that the AZ vaccine would also be ineffective against Delta, given it was an old-fashioned vaccine (as opposed to the mRNA options) that could only target the original Wuhan strain. It did not help that AZ showed early signs of side effects that could lead to blood clots. This was rare, but the news created fears about vaccine safety.

I was concerned about AZ and went public with my advice that patients should pass on it until the mRNA vaccines, due to arrive shortly, were available. Some took my advice; some didn't. The mRNA vaccines were indeed preferable, both in effectiveness and safety. The Pfizer-BioNTech and Moderna mRNA versions were clinically similar, yet brand loyalties developed and became a focus of conversation—"Which shot did you get?"

It was becoming politically difficult to continue locking down and keeping measures like border restrictions in place. Conspiracy theories were everywhere, creating real barriers to vaccinating the last quintile of the population. In Alberta, Premier Jason Kenney had a particularly rough ride: his United Conservative Party split over the need to restrict individual freedoms (never mind that most of the country thought he should be doing a lot more), eventually ending his career.[37]

Canada escaped the third wave with relatively fewer deaths: 4,375 succumbed to infection this time thanks to a relatively high vaccine uptake rate of 80 percent.[38] But it didn't feel much better. Hospitals and ICU units had once again hit capacity. Even with another summer on the horizon, the pandemic continued to take its toll, physically, emotionally, socially, economically, and politically. And new variants kept emerging, with the most contagious—Omicron—still to come.

Wave Four

When case counts rose in the late summer of 2021, governments employed various measures to increase the number of vaccinated citizens. The federal government, various provinces, cities, universities, and private companies gave employees the choice between getting vaccinated and getting terminated. In September, Ontario became the fourth province to introduce a "vaccine passport" (all but Nunavut would eventually do so). These passports became de facto necessities if one wanted to participate in public life.[39] Restaurant personnel were among those tasked with checking the passports of customers, forcing them into the unwelcome role of pandemic social police.

By fall 2021, boosters were recommended to most people under the age of sixty-five, who were asked to get their booster six months after their last dose or infection. People at high risk of severe COVID-19 illness were strongly advised to get their booster at a three-month interval to provide optimal protection.[40] The advice was not always taken. Vaccine fatigue was becoming a factor. While four in five Canadians received their first two doses, far fewer lined up for boosters.[41]

The fault lines in public opinion on vaccines were by now well established. To the antivaxx contingent, mandates and vaccine passports seemed like a totalitarian "papers please" imposition on their personal liberties. To most others, the vaccination requirement was a simple and reasonable way to allow people to live relatively normal lives while we were still in the midst of a destructive pandemic. The two sides seemed to live in entirely different worlds and the passport program, regardless of its merits (which were many), served to separate them further. Many families and friends were torn apart over this issue.

Wave Five

As Christmas 2021 approached, it appeared another lockdown would be necessary, but many were now done with COVID-19. Several people I know in Toronto took off to jurisdictions such as Florida where, from a public policy perspective, the pandemic was over and they could live without restrictions. But Omicron was here[42] and while it was less fatal, it was virulently contagious.

In January 2022, Ontario entered a partial lockdown (termed as a rollback to "Step 2" of the previous roadmap) due to record Omicron cases. Most non-essential indoor facilities were ordered closed. It was the lightest and briefest lockdown of the bunch, yet it was the one that pushed many over the edge. The Freedom Convoy would roll into Ottawa in a matter of weeks. By the time it rolled out, with help from several police forces, it was clear to governments all over Canada that sweeping social controls were no longer feasible. Some restrictions lingered on, particularly in COVID hotspots, but we were through with lockdowns.

Ontario had not only the longest lockdown in Canada but the longest in North America. According to Dan Kelly, CEO of the Canadian Federation of Independent Business, it was the longest lockdown in the world.[43] The goodwill that had marked the early stages of the pandemic in March 2020 had by then entirely evaporated, a victim of some mix of fatigue, government overreach, and the corrosive effects of misinformation and dishonesty.

Waves Six, Seven, and Beyond

More waves followed in spring and summer of 2022, although they got significantly less press as the era of lockdowns was over. Now, we rarely hear about a "wave" of COVID-19, even with the virus still circulating.

There are almost certainly more waves to come. The updated bivalent vaccine boosters of 2022 were very helpful in addressing Omicron strains 1 and 2, but they were not as effective as the initial batch, simply because it has been difficult to pin down a dominant strain derived from the original Omicron variant. According to the National Institute of Health (NIH), the bivalent booster vaccines against SARS-CoV-2 were 37 percent more effective than older booster shots at reducing the risk of severe COVID-19.[44] The increased protection against hospitalization or death was seen regardless of age or whether people had previously received a different booster.

I've seen an outbreak of COVID-19 infections among some of my patients in March 2023, but these folks have been fully vaccinated and have come through their infection without much issue and did not need Paxlovid. As of March 2023, the dominant variant is XBB.1.5, comprising 89.6 percent of cases, followed by BQ.1.1, with 6.7 percent of cases. "The original Omicron variant is gone now," says infectious disease expert Dr. Mark Rupp. "Currently subvariants of Omicron are circulating, including XBB.1.5, BQ.1.1 and BQ.1."[45]

On March 3, 2023, Health Canada was encouraging people at high risk to get yet another bivalent booster.[46] I had to ask myself, "Why?". If the vaccine is no longer genetically close to the most current strains, a booster would be even less effective than in spring 2022. This is yet another public service announcement that seems to me destined to further erode the credibility of public health. Maybe they assume no one checks the science or, worse, that no one cares.

To date, I've had a total of four vaccine doses. I was infected with Omicron in the early days of December 2021, but followed up to get my bivalent six months later. For now, my thinking is, "if I am fully vaccinated, let the descendants of Omicron come to get me." At this stage, infection will likely lead to a better natural immunity option than an outdated bivalent booster that focused on Omicron 1. But let me be professionally correct by saying you should talk to your health-care professional to determine if a bivalent vaccine booster is right for you.

CHAPTER TWO

THE HEALTH CONSEQUENCES OF COVID-19

As the title of this book suggests, we are all still sick, even those of us who survived COVID-19 or never even contracted it. We are still feeling the effects of the pandemic, whether or not we want to admit it. Maybe we have the lingering effects of a COVID-19 infection called Long COVID, or vaccine side effects, or we're still feeling the psychological and social impacts of lockdowns and isolation. No one has been spared. The trauma was both individual and collective.

As of March 2023, the official number of COVID-19 cases confirmed by the World Health Organization globally was around 760 million people, with almost 103 million in the United States and 4.5 million in Canada. Note that the WHO refers to "confirmed cases". This means that a test needed to be completed in a lab (to be official); it had to be positive; and it had to be recorded by a public health entity which then reported it back to the WHO's global dashboard. The official count is almost certainly too low, and possibly ridiculously so.

Many of us have experienced testing negative on a COVID-19 PCR test despite exhibiting all the signs and symptoms of a COVID-19 infection. This is called a false negative result. While PCR testing is both sensitive and specific, the test needs to sample enough viral load to become positive. As well, some people tested positive and did not report the result, or got sick and didn't bother testing because they could not access a test or decided the outcome would not change because there was no real treatment. They were locked down with nowhere to spread it.

A Bloomberg article in June 2022 asked readers if they felt "gaslighted" by the total official case count. People seemed to think the reported numbers were far too low. No one knows for sure what the multiplier is for total versus reported cases. Shockingly, some studies suggest a range of three times to thirty times.[1]

Another June 2022 survey in the US led researchers to believe that more than 40 percent of adults reported having COVID-19 and nearly one in five of those (19 percent) were currently still experiencing symptoms of Long COVID, which we will discuss later.[2] Furthermore, I discovered within my own practice that almost 40 percent of our patients who tested positive for COVID-19 antibodies were surprised. Many assured me they didn't have any symptoms. This finding meant that many infections were asymptomatic.

Obviously, the most serious consequence of COVID-19 was the death toll. Some were "lucky" to have succumbed relatively quickly. They would progress from feeling fine to developing a high fever and being unable to breathe in a matter of hours. Often in these cases, the patient would go to the emergency department, be admitted to hospital, and pass away in a matter of days. The immediate cause of death would be sudden multi-organ failure triggered by COVID-19. The virus ravaged every tissue in the body.

Any infection such as COVID-19 can cause the body to mount a response to fight it off. The body releases a chain of reactions that can range from creating heat—what we call a fever—to producing mucus in our nose and lungs to flush out the virus, which is why we get runny noses and cough up phlegm when we're sick. Various types of white blood cells attack tissues infected with the virus. This causes local areas to become red and swollen—we call that inflammation.

Unfortunately, sometimes the body can mount an overactive response that causes inflammation throughout the body, leading to aches and pains. Sometimes, in more serious cases, other organs are involved. All of this happens while the body begins to manufacture antibodies over several days to lock down and remove the virus. Most of the time, the organ tissue recovers by renewing itself, but if the inflammatory response is especially intense, there can be unintended consequences. Lungs drown in fluid from the mucus being produced. The heart beats irregularly due to damaged electrical circuits in the heart tissues. Hence, the heart cannot produce enough blood pressure to oxygenate tissues. Meanwhile, the liver and kidneys cannot filter the massive amount of toxins. Acute multi-organ failure can be a fast and less painful death for the patient, if not for their families.

Less fortunate patients suffered a slow death with a full presence of mind. They entered the hospital with some shortness of breath and, given their low oxygenation and confirmation that they have COVID-19 pneumonia, were admitted. As their hospital stays continued, things deteriorated. Early in the pandemic, COVID-19 patients did not respond to the limited medications available. Most of the drugs were for support, such as Ventolin to open up airways and diuretics to reduce water in the lungs. None of the known anti-virals were working. Even worse, the drugs used to treat the fever would sometimes work together with the virus to make the kidney and liver work too hard. The drugs can often increase organ function, but in a scenario with organ inflammation caused by the virus, it leads to more acute organ damage. On it goes. The body uses its antibodies to fight a losing battle against the virus as doctors and nurses can do nothing but comfort the patient and watch.

Most patients who had pre-existing issues like heart, lung, or kidney disease had a poor outcome because they were not fit enough to do battle. Those with borderline diabetes or diabetes saw their blood sugar increase; a normal reaction to any illness as the body gives its organs fuel to fight. But this fuel was good for the virus, too. As the organs failed, the virus won and the patient died a slow version of the multi-organ death I described above. Patients and families had time to choose whether to go on a ventilator or not. And say goodbye to family.

As of March 31, 2023, statistics from the World Health Organization showed that 52,000 Canadians and 1.1 million Americans succumbed to the virus. Globally, the death toll is around 7 million people.[3]

Statistics can be impersonal and sterile. Think about it this way. The equivalent of 288 Airbus 320 planeloads of Canadians perished in three years (180 passengers/plane).[4] Sixteen Super Bowl stadiums full of Americans perished (70,000 fans/stadium)[5] The entire population of Arizona (7.4 million) was lost globally.[6]

* * *

Those numbers may not be accurate. It is neat-and-tidy to think we can tabulate COVID-19 deaths simply according to death certificates that list COVID-19 as the specific cause of death. But data scientists have identified an excess of mortality during the pandemic that tells another story.

Experts anticipate that there will always be some degree of variation in the overall number of deaths recorded from week to week and year to year. The variations, however, are fairly consistent; they occur within a certain range established by historical and demographic trends. Unfortunately, the pandemic data reveals more deaths than expected throughout the pandemic and the increase is far outside of the established range, even once deaths attributed directly to COVID-19 are backed out. It is probable that we have seriously undercounted deaths as well as infections.

Canada experienced 40,349 deaths in excess of expectations from March 2020 to the middle of February 2022. That is an increase of 7.4 percent over what would normally be expected in that time frame. Within this period, 32,490 reported deaths were directly attributed to COVID-19.[7] That leaves just under 8,000 excess deaths unexplained.

Notably, the greatest excess of deaths occurred from around December 2021 to the end of January 2022, when the extremely infectious Omicron variant was dominant. Omicron was less deadly than previous variants on a per capita basis, but because more people became sick, more deaths resulted. Overall, the total number of deaths swelled from 30,866 in December 2021 to 35,125 in January 2022, an increase of 13.8 percent. The expected increase from one month to the other, if there were no pandemic, would have been around 5.5 percent.[8]

It was widely assumed that deaths increased primarily among seniors. While the elderly disproportionately account for much of the overall pandemic death toll, the trends in excess mortality were observed across all age groups and, in fact, younger Canadians were well represented.

The forty-five-and-under age group accounted for just over 15 percent more deaths than expected in January 2022; those over the age of forty-five accounted for approximately 13 percent more deaths than expected.[9] Higher vaccination rates among the elderly population may help to explain this surprising finding.

There were also notable gender differences in the excess mortality rate. In January 2022, approximately 12 percent more deaths were attributed to males than females (6 percent). There were also regional differences. In Alberta, deaths among males increased by 23.6 percent compared with females at 15.7 percent and in British Columbia, deaths among males increased by 26.5 percent compared with females at 16.6 percent. In all provinces, the least vaccinated adult age group was those under thirty.[10] Females took the vaccine more than males. British Columbians were the least vaccinated in Canada.[11]

Canada was not alone in its excess mortality. While the official number of US COVID-19 deaths since the start of the pandemic is 1.1 million, the Centers for Disease Control and Prevention have identified an additional 300,000 excess American deaths over the past three years. As in Canada, most of this excess mortality has been attributed to COVID-19 (roughly 25 percent was due to other causes).[12]

The *Economist* has calculated the mortality caused by the pandemic in the United States to be 20 percent higher than its official COVID-19 death toll. A different Centers for Disease Control and Prevention (CDC) data set suggests an excess of only about 10 percent (which is still more than 100,000 people). Other models see excesses of 15 percent and some as high as 50 percent.[13]

Harvard University professors Jeremy Faust and Benjy Renton found their American data on the excess deaths to be an almost perfect match with the peaks and troughs of the COVID-19 death curve, which supports the idea that the excess is pandemic related.[14]

In the US, as elsewhere, there were delays in health-care delivery during the pandemic, but this does not appear to account for many of the excess deaths. The delays were mostly early on. Health care services largely resumed as normal after 2020. The incidence of a pattern of excess of deaths during and after 2020 looks much the same. Also, CDC data suggests an increase of only about 28,000 "above average" deaths from cancer during the full pandemic,[15] a small fraction of the excess mortality. Accidental and nonmedical deaths such as those attributed to car crashes, homicide, suicide, and overdoses represented barely 5 percent of excess mortality, according to Harvard's Dr. Faust.

Faust argues that if Long COVID and its sequelae (re-infections) from COVID-19 were responsible for increasing excess mortality, it should show up as a spike after each wave of the pandemic peaks. It doesn't. He concludes that we have likely under-counted COVID-19 deaths. It is probable that people died at home from COVID-19 and were never properly recorded in the COVID-19 statistics, especially if no tests were conducted to show a positive diagnosis. Faust's analysis indicates more excess deaths in the early days of the pandemic, when testing was difficult to access and the dominant virus strain was more deadly. "I suspect, in the fullness of time," he says, "we're going to figure out that of these 200,000 to 300,000 excess deaths, that 80 to 90 percent of them were just COVID."[16]

I do not doubt that Canada under-counted deaths due to COVID-19. It was far more difficult to access testing here than in the US, especially early in the pandemic with the simple lack of testing capacity and the need for scheduling appointments.[17] Many who died, especially in more rural communities, did not know they had COVID-19.

* * *

Beyond under-counting deaths directly caused by COVID-19, what else could account for all the excess deaths of Canadians, Americans, and Europeans during the height of the pandemic waves? There are several hypotheses.

One is widespread "failure to thrive." The National Institute on Aging describes failure to thrive as "a syndrome of weight loss, decreased appetite and poor nutrition and inactivity, often accompanied by dehydration, depressive symptoms, impaired immune function, and low cholesterol."

In the early days of the pandemic, we witnessed a disproportionate death rate amongst seniors, many of whom were in nursing or retirement homes and were already frail, not to mention unvaccinated. These places were fertile ground for the early, more deadly strains of the virus. Seniors succumbed to infection in droves. The institutions in which they lived were not equipped to manage the spread of sickness. Caregivers themselves became infected and spread the virus. As documented earlier, many seniors were not given proper care, largely due to staffing shortfalls or poor training and lapsed standards. Some were denied even the basics of water and food, and died tragic, lonely, and painful deaths of malnutrition and dehydration. Their death certificates may not say they died of COVID-19, but their deaths may well have resulted from it.

Many people suffered and are still dealing with lingering effects that health-care professionals define as Long COVID or "Post COVID-19 Syndrome." These, too, could account for excess death.

"Post-COVID-19 syndrome involves a variety of new, returning or ongoing symptoms that people experience more than four weeks after getting COVID-19," writes the Mayo Clinic. "In some people, post-COVID-19 syndrome lasts months or years or causes disability."[18] Among the symptoms: fatigue, which can worsen after physical or mental effort; neurological issues including difficulty thinking or concentrating, headache, sleep problems, dizziness, pins-and-needles sensation, and loss of taste or smell); respiratory problems, including difficulty breathing or shortness of breath and coughing; joint or muscle pain; heart issues, including chest pain and a rapid or pounding heartbeat; digestive problems, including diarrhea and cramping pain; skin rash; mental health issues, including depressed mood and anxiety. Symptoms can occur as soon as one month or longer after having COVID-19.

The incidence of Long Covid is higher than you might think. An October 2022 study from Statistics Canada found that 15 percent of Canadians who had contracted COVID-19 were still suffering from symptoms consistent with Long COVID.[19] This study was based on the experiences of nearly 100,000 patients and revealed worrisome evidence that many people have not fully recovered several months after being infected.[20] The study found one in twenty had not recovered and 42 percent reported only a partial recovery between six and eighteen months after infection.

More recent 2022 global data suggests almost half of COVID-19 survivors report persistent symptoms four months after their diagnosis.[21] The prevalence of Long COVID is around 43 percent and the range can vary from 9 percent to 81 percent due to differences in sex, region, and study population.[22] The risk of Long COVID associated with the Delta variant appears to be higher when compared to the Omicron variant.[23]

As one would expect, those who were hospitalized with the virus were far more likely to experience Long COVID (54 percent compared to only 34 percent of outpatients). Also, the unvaccinated appear to have it worst. A 2021 survey showed that more than 90 percent of the 3,700 participants who had COVID-19 without the benefit of vaccines reported a recovery time exceeding thirty-five weeks. By month six, most still reported fatigue, malaise, and cognitive dysfunction.[24]

It can be difficult to tell whether these symptoms are specifically due to COVID-19 or are an exacerbation of pre-existing medical conditions. The virus does tend to exacerbate things. It became apparent early in the pandemic that people with pre-existing physical conditions such as heart disease, diabetes, cancer, and asthma were at higher risk of serious complications and death if they contracted COVID-19.[25] It also appears that the virus can trigger entirely new problems.

It has been demonstrated that some people who suffered severe cases of COVID-19 experience new "multiorgan effects or autoimmune conditions with symptoms lasting weeks, months, or even years after" their original illness.[26] These are the result of the super-inflammatory response I mentioned above, an overly aggressive effort of the body to rid the virus. It can result in permanent tissue damage and scarring of the body's organs. This may be how Long COVID accounts for some portion of the excess deaths.

Many COVID patients who wound up in intensive care units technically beat the infection but developed these other problems. In one Manitoba study, less than 8 percent of ICU patients were still testing positive after thirteen days in the hospital. By around day twenty-five, the viral load had become undetectable.[27] Yet some patients remained in the ICU, not because of the viral load but because they continued to experience organ failure due to acute and intense inflammation in the early days of their infection.

It should be obvious, given that COVID-19 is a respiratory infection, that some amount of lung damage would be evident in patients post-infection. Indeed, an October 2022 United Kingdom study concluded approximately 11 percent of COVID-19 patients develop interstitial lung disease after hospitalization.[28] For some, this lung damage resolves, but for others, it appears to lead to a progression of lung fibrosis.

Simply put, fibrosis is scarring. After a significant amount of damage due to COVID-19 pneumonia, the tissues of the lung stiffen or fibrose, making breathing more difficult because the lungs are no longer able to expand and collapse easily to exchange gases (oxygen in, carbon dioxide out). Such an outcome worsens the patient's quality of life and decreases life expectancy. With weaker lungs, it is far easier to develop pneumonia with any respiratory infection. Scientists have also noted that our immune system weakens after infection and even more so after reinfection, leading to other non-COVID causes of death such as bacterial or other viral infections, including pneumonia.[29]

Cardiologists have now recognized that the risk of cardiovascular problems such as a heart attack or stroke can remain heightened for many months even after a full recovery from a COVID-19 infection. As one might expect, patients who were admitted to intensive care with acute infections had a twenty-fold higher risk of cardiovascular problems such as congestive heart failure and DVT (deep vein thrombosis, or blood clots), when compared with the uninfected. Even those who had not been hospitalized had increased risks of a variety of heart conditions, ranging from an 8 percent increase in the rate of heart attacks to a 247 percent increase in the rate of heart inflammation.[30]

Blood vessels can also become inflamed, which increases the risk of atherosclerosis—the narrowing and hardening of the arteries. When they get to a critical narrow width, blood cannot easily flow through the arteries, and heart attacks and strokes can occur. Clotting can also happen. When this occurs in the veins, we call it a DVT. The most dangerous complications of DVTs are when a part of the clot breaks off and travels through the bloodstream to the lungs, causing a blockage known as a pulmonary embolism. Even a small pulmonary embolism can damage the lungs and a large one can be fatal.

Researchers are just beginning to learn about COVID's impact on parts of the brain.[31] Forty percent of recovered COVID-19 patients showed material changes in their brains, specifically in the white matter and brainstem. Changes in our white matter can lead to fatigue, insomnia, anxiety, depression, headaches, and cognitive problems. Brainstem changes can impact our circadian rhythm control, which can lead to sleep problems. We'll talk more about this in the next chapter.

The kidneys are not spared in the acute and post-acute phases of COVID-19 infection. Patients displayed a lower glomerular filtration rate, meaning kidney function had become suboptimal. Technically, how sick you were with COVID-19 determined the severity of acute kidney injury (AKI).[32] Unfortunately, the kidney does not regenerate its tissues, unlike the liver and some other organs. It houses many delicate filters that act as a recycling system. Once these fine filters get damaged from inflammation and scarring, the kidney no longer functions efficiently. Treatment may then include dialysis and, hopefully, a successful kidney transplant. Unfortunately, some Long COVID-19 patients do succumb to kidney failure.

Here's yet another hypothesis that may account for some of the excess deaths. In a massive study of over 200,000 patients, researchers at the Veterans Affairs St. Louis Healthcare System in Missouri found those who had been infected with even a mild COVID-19 infection had a greater risk of developing diabetes.[33] People who caught the virus were 40 percent more likely than veterans in the control group to develop diabetes up to a year after infection. Those with a high body mass index (BMI) doubled their chances of developing diabetes in the year after.[34]

Two of the most common forms of diabetes are type I, largely a genetic condition that manifests early in a person's life, and type II, which is related to a person's lifestyle. You are more likely to develop type II diabetes if you are overweight and physically inactive, hence the increased risk of people with a high body mass index (BMI). We know that type II diabetes is largely due to an insufficiency in the pancreas: in simple terms, this organ does not make enough insulin to reduce blood sugar levels. It is not difficult to see how a pancreas weakened by COVID-19 infection and damaged by inflammation can set a person up for the onset of diabetes months or years later. While diabetes does not directly kill the patient, we know diabetes causes inflammation of the arteries and later, atherosclerosis (hardening of the arteries). Diabetes kills indirectly by increasing one's risk of heart attack, stroke, and kidney failure.

* * *

Yet another hypothesis is that delayed care contributed to the excess of deaths. There is ample evidence that many people had their needed medical care postponed, including screening procedures, annual check-ups, or routine follow-ups of medical conditions. Delayed cancer screenings and cancer care, in particular, are already leading to much worse diagnoses and prognoses than patients would otherwise have received. Early cancer screening, such as mammograms, colonoscopies, or pap smears, saves lives because an early-stage cancer diagnosis can lead to more timely care and a more curative outcome or prolonged survival. Unfortunately, many people chose to delay their screenings, often because fear and anxiety over COVID-19 overwhelmed their willingness to do something they may have felt was not medically urgent. Others had their screenings pushed back because hospital resources were refocused on suppressing the pandemic Breast cancer screenings dropped by around 90 percent and colorectal cancer screenings by about 85 percent through May 2020.[35]

As a result of decreased screening, the incidences of new cancer diagnoses dropped. For example, new lung cancer diagnoses decreased by 47 percent and new melanoma diagnoses dropped by 67 percent in spring 2020 compared with 2019.[36] The Ontario Canada health database found a similar 41 percent decrease in breast, cervical, and lung cancer screening in 2020 compared to 2019.[37] To be clear, cancer did not stop growing in people—we were just not finding it.

By July 2020, the United States saw an increase in screening rates, but they were still 29 to 36 percent lower than pre-COVID-19 levels. By March 2021, breast cancer screening rose to levels that were 13 percent below historical averages, while colon cancer and cervical cancer screenings rose to 25 percent below the average values.[38] Canada experienced a cancer screening level that was 20 to 35 percent below pre-pandemic levels as of January 2021.[39]

Delays in screening resulted in delayed diagnoses. Data from the Washington State Surveillance, Epidemiology, and End Results (SEER) registry showed a lower increase of stage 1 colorectal cancer (small and highly treatable) during the early and later phases of the pandemic, yet an increased incidence of stage IV cases of colorectal cancer (advanced or metastatic, meaning it has spread to other organs or parts of the body) over the same period.[40]

In the United States, The National Cancer Institute estimates a 1 percent increase in breast and colorectal cancer deaths over the next ten years, which translates to 10,000 excess deaths as a result of delayed screening and treatment.[41] The National Health Service (NHS) in the United Kingdom estimated an 8 to 9.5 percent increase in deaths from breast cancer because of a later-stage diagnosis.

Those who were diagnosed with cancer just before the pandemic faced severe disruptions to their care due to reduced hospital capacity and concerns over their susceptibility to the serious risks of COVID-19. While the official directive of all hospitals was to continue all urgent care, the reality was that their capacity was very limited.[42] What had been routinely operable or treatable before became more complicated, if not deadly.

The Lancet Oncology reported in 2020 that "a five to 10 percent decrease in survival in high-income countries has been predicted, which will account for hundreds of thousands of excess deaths, dwarfing those caused by COVID-19."[43]

Of course, cancer screenings weren't the only things we delayed. Heart bypass surgeries (CABG) were pushed back, potentially leading to unnecessary heart attacks. MRI scans, already in short supply, were especially difficult to access, causing setbacks in diagnostic and treatment decisions. The average Canadian was waiting 5.4 weeks for a computed tomography (CT) scan, 10.6 weeks for a magnetic resonance imaging (MRI) scan, and 4.9 weeks for an ultrasound in 2022.[44] People who have experienced mobility and visual impairment will suffer longer as they wait for corrective surgeries, such as joint replacements and eye surgeries.

In the midst of the pandemic, it seemed reasonable to pause the routine annual screening, and diagnosis and treatment of symptoms and conditions not considered medically urgent, or at least less urgent than COVID-19. In retrospect, we clearly should not have sacrificed diagnostics and treatments for so long.

The Canadian health-care system is in worse shape now because of the pandemic, but the data tells us that it was already in distress before COVID-19. The virus simply pushed it over the edge. For thirty years, the Fraser Institute has surveyed specialist physicians across twelve specialties and ten provinces. Its 2022 report included data collected from January 10 to September 15, 2022. Researchers revealed a median waiting time of 27.4 weeks (6.4 months or half a year!) between a referral from a general practitioner and receipt of treatment. Before the pandemic, this same wait was 25.6 weeks, so we've now gone from bad to dreadful. This most recent wait time is the longest recorded in this survey's history; an eye-popping 195 percent longer than in 1993, when it was "only" 9.3 weeks or under three months.[45]

Physicians consider a reasonable wait time between consultation and treatment to be no longer than eight weeks (excluding limb or life-threatening treatments).[46] We now have 1.2 million Canadians on waiting lists for at least one procedure dating from 2022 and almost all of them will wait far longer than that. Waiting for treatment has now become the defining characteristic of Canadian health care for the average Canadian.

As we've seen with cancer, delays in treatment have serious consequences. They lead to poorer medical outcomes, whether it's increased pain and suffering, physical disabilities, or seeing potentially reversible illnesses or injuries turn into chronic or irreversible conditions, resulting in permanent disabilities and premature death. Some patients have had to stop working and sacrifice their wages while they wait for their consultation and/or treatment, causing financial hardship for patients and their families.

Mental distress is yet another consideration. The fear and worry of waiting for a specialist weighed on many Canadians during the pandemic, adding to an already enormous load of emotional and mental distress, a subject to which we'll turn next.

Screening and treatment delays created downstream issues that will continue to impact the health-care system for many years to come. They help to explain why so many people are still not feeling right after they've technically beaten COVID and, in my view, they are also one of the silent killers of the pandemic, accounting for some of the deaths in excess of expectations.

CHAPTER THREE

LOCKDOWNS AND MENTAL HEALTH

Lockdowns and social restrictions were extraordinary, unprecedented responses to a public health hazard. You'll recall that we were initially told the lockdowns would last two weeks. If that had been all of it, we likely would have suffered less in the way of adverse consequences to mental health. But the lockdowns kept coming. They differed from province to province and wave to wave and not everyone adhered to the rules, but restrictions kept the vast majority of people indoors and isolated for long periods for over two years. What had begun as a temporary emergency measure evolved into a way of life. We subjected entire populations to massive experiments in acute social deprivation and disruption without forethought or planning.

It's worth noting that our collective mental health was not great going into the pandemic. We know that in any given year, one in five people battle with a mental health issue.[1] We have insufficient resources to manage mental health at the best of times, let alone when we add an explosive, additional burden on top. The results have been alarming. Millions of people have been broken regardless of whether or not they were ever infected by COVID-19.

There is no end to science demonstrating that human beings are social animals. The best predictor of physical health and well-being, as well as fertility and longevity, is a person's close friendships and relationships. The frequency of social interactions also predicts a person's feelings of happiness and contentment and trust in his or her community. We like to be able to see one another and be close to one another—it's built into our endorphin system. Relationships are crucial to mental health. Indeed, all of our culture and everything we consider important to civilization is dependent on our social relationships.[2]

The seemingly endless stream of lockdowns and restrictions on social gatherings severely interfered with human relations. Unfortunately, the pandemic came at a time when we were already fairly isolated, at least relative to previous generations. More of us are living on our own today: 4.4 million Canadians.[3] Three in ten of our households are solo. That means we depend more than we have historically on the workplace and our communities for social interaction. The pandemic brought those occasions to a screeching halt.

While there isn't much literature on the impact of mass isolation, primarily because we don't make a habit of it, the effects of isolation on individuals are well documented. A summary of the research in a 2017 article noted demonstrable associations between loneliness and depression, suicidal behaviour, personality disorders, and psychoses. "Among people with severe mental illness," it added, "social isolation has been linked to higher levels of delusions, lack of insight, and high hospital usage. Conversely, people who report greater informal social support have been found more likely to recover from psychotic symptoms."[4]

There have also been a number of large studies on social deprivation among seniors and the results are not good: it reduces cognitive capacity and the sense of physical and mental well-being, not to mention longevity. Chronic isolation risks depression and dementia and has also been associated with higher risks of cardiovascular disease and cancer.

We are not meant to be alone.

A UK study carried out during the pandemic confirms that lockdowns elevated levels of anxiety and depression, reduced physical activity, increased feelings of loneliness, increased instances of suicide ideation, and generally harmed mental health. People who met the clinical criteria for anxiety, depression, and post-traumatic stress disorder reported twice the rates of loneliness as the rest of the population. People who were lonely had more trouble maintaining emotional regulation and sleep patterns.

All of these effects tended to be exacerbated by low levels of physical exertion and a lot of sitting around.

The science shows that women, and young women in particular, tend to invest more in their social circles than men, maintaining more close friendships and more emotionally intense relationships. It is no wonder, then, that they were hit particularly hard during COVID, experiencing higher overall levels of distress, panic, and depression. New data shows that if you also suffered from Long COVID, you are still more likely to develop symptoms of mental disorders.

A major study in *Nature* enumerated the consequences of the lockdowns once they were in progress and concluded that they are "likely to have demonstrable mental health and psychosocial ramifications for years to come. This will inevitably place a significant burden on our health system and societies."

It continues: "Worryingly, prolonged social isolation seems to invoke changes in the capacity to visualize internally centred thoughts, especially in younger sub-population. This may presage a switch from an outward to an inward focus that may exacerbate the experience of social isolation in susceptible individuals."

Worse still, as the same study notes, social isolation is known to have significant effects on the structure and function of the hippocampus and default network, long recognized as a primary neural pathway implicated in dementia and other major neurodegenerative diseases: "The fact that these same brain regions turn up in the neuroanatomical consequences of COVID-19 infection is concerning."

And, sadly, the study finds that social inequality affected the impact of the pandemic and that the negative outcomes from COVID-19 fall disproportionately on "families of lower socio-economic status, single-parent households, and those with racial and ethnic minority backgrounds." We put the most stress on our most vulnerable.

* * *

There were warning signs very early in the pandemic. In April 2020, an American survey found 41 percent of respondents reported at least one adverse mental or behavioral health condition during social restrictions. Symptoms of anxiety disorder or depressive disorder registered at 30.9 percent. Symptoms of trauma and stressor-related disorder (TSRD) related to the pandemic were at 26.3 percent.

That was only one month after the pandemic was announced and before the initial sense of we're-all-in-this-together broke down under cascading case counts and frustrations over the relentlessness of the virus and lockdowns. At the height of the pandemic in early 2021, symptoms consistent with anxiety and depression were reported by four in ten American adults; more than three in ten were still reporting symptoms in early 2023. Some people were more likely to be troubled than others. Five in ten of those who experienced household job loss reported symptoms of anxiety and depression. Perhaps counter-intuitively, given that the elderly were most at risk, only two in ten adults over age sixty-five had these symptoms while five in ten of the eighteen-to-twenty-four cohort did. Rates of persistent feelings of hopelessness and sadness were 20 percent higher among high-school age women during the pandemic than before it began.

The World Health Organization announced last year that during the first year of the pandemic, the prevalence of anxiety and depression increased 25 percent worldwide. Again, the leading stressors were grief, loneliness, and financial worries, along with fear of infection and fear for the well-being of loved ones. And, again, young people and women were disproportionately affected, along with people who had pre-existing physical conditions such as asthma, cancer, and heart disease. "The information we have now about the impact of COVID-19 on the world's mental health is just the tip of the iceberg," said Dr. Tedros Adhanom Ghebreyesus, WHO director-general. "This is a wake-up call to all countries to pay more attention to mental health and do a better job of supporting their populations' mental health."[5]

In the middle of the pandemic, Canada's public health agency reported numbers higher than the WHO's global data and more in line with the US experience. Between February and May 2021, four in ten Canadians reported distress, most commonly feelings of anxiety and depression, but also agitation and lack of energy. The incidence of anxiety and depression was highest among those aged eighteen to thirty-four, especially women. One notable difference from the US survey is that Canadian women over the age of sixty-five also reported high levels of anxiety and depression. Front-line workers, those who saw their incomes affected, and those who suffered loss were also disproportionately struggling.[6]

Not surprisingly, Canadian's mental health appears to have continued to deteriorate as the pandemic wore on. In 2022, an Angus Reid Institute/CBC survey found that 54 percent of Canadians said their mental health had worsened in the first two years of COVID. Women aged thirty-five to fifty-four were the highest at 63 percent, followed closely by women aged eighteen to thirty-four at 60 percent.

All of this shed light on a recent report from the insurance firm Sun Life. It found that one in three Canadians reported severe symptoms of burnout during the pandemic. Drug claim data demonstrate that requests for mental health medications went through the roof in the period 2019 to 2021, with claimants under the age of thirty-five leading the way.[7]

It appears that many of the ill effects people suffered during the pandemic ended or were reduced at the lifting of restrictions. In March 2023, a group of researchers led by McGill University and including collaborators from McMaster, the University of Toronto, and other institutions, reviewed almost 140 papers dealing with reported mental health issues in adults, children, and adolescents between the ages of ten to nineteen. While self-reported data in 2021 suggested significant and long-lasting mental health challenges with COVID-related issues like illness, vaccine hesitancy, financial insecurity, loss of social engagement, and access to health services,[8] people appear to have come out the other side stronger than initially feared. Depression symptoms worsened minimally in older adults, university students, and people who self-identified as belonging to a sexual or gender minority group. Women experienced more anxiety, depression, and generally poorer mental health. Only small studies found these symptoms worse among parents. The review concluded that there are limited lingering impacts on the mental health of people from middle to high-income countries and no changes were found for general mental health or anxiety symptoms or suicide rates.[9]

* * *

It is important to note that public health measures were not the only factors messing with people's minds during the pandemic. Politics also mattered. There has been a palpable feeling of negativity, anger, and rage around the world over the last three years. It feels as though the proverbial global temperature turned way up. Of course, it had been reported well before COVID-19 that we were seeing a broad shattering of societal norms and an embrace of extremes through the Trump years, and it is easy to overestimate the level of anger in society when the most extreme statements and personalities are favoured by social media algorithms. But there's evidence that the relentlessly bleak news stories of the past few years had an effect.

Pollara Insights published a "Rage Index" in August 2022. It is meant to measure "the mood of Canadians regarding their governments, the economy, and current events."[10] That we even need something called a "Rage Index" is a troubling sign of the times, but now that it exists, it gives us a snapshot of the modern psyche. Fortunately, the number of Canadians who report feeling "very angry" about the government, recent news, societal changes, the economy, and their personal finances is still in the low double digits, hitting a high of 17 percent regarding the economy.

However, once the "very angry" are combined with those who are feeling "annoyed or moderately angry," we see that the majority of Canadians (60 percent) are implicated. Perhaps worse, only 5 percent of us consider ourselves "very happy." Less than 10 percent consider ourselves either "very happy" or "pleased, moderately happy, or very happy" about the direction Canada is headed. The same goes for the state of our economy. Less than 5 percent are any level of pleased or happy about what they are reading in the news. And while a third of us are pleased, moderately happy, or very happy with the state of our personal finances, less than 10 percent feel that way about the direction of the Canadian economy. The Pollara researchers conclude that Canadians are broadly grumpy but intense rage is limited to a vocal minority. A *very* vocal minority.[11]

The Rage Index captures something about how the pandemic and politics and our feelings about them are related. The state of our economic life is also relevant: it was massively disrupted by the pandemic. Whereas the Rage Index is a new tool, with no year-over-year or historical comparisons available, the Misery Index has been used to evaluate the state of the economy and its impact on societies for over fifty years.

Initially known by the less catchy title Economic Discomfort Index, the Misery Index was created by economist Arthur Okun in the 1960s. It combines the unemployment rate and the inflation rate. Although it is rare for both unemployment and inflation to be high at the same time, there have been instances of this occurring, notably during the episodes of stagflation in the 1970s.[12] Inflation was over 8 percent in North America in June 2022, and the Misery Index reached a relatively high rate of 12.6 percent.[13] Even when subtracting peak months, as Bloomberg Economics did during the pandemic crisis in early 2020, the index still sat at around 12 percent. This represents the highest levels seen in over a decade, rivaling the aftermath of the Great Recession when then-President Barack Obama oversaw an unemployment rate of around 10 percent.[14] In Canada, the Misery Index sat at 13 percent in May 2022—the highest in almost thirty years.[15]

When you add political rage and economic misery to the challenges of the pandemic, it's no wonder we're feeling sad, angry, and even a little crazy. As this book was going to press, a Kaiser Foundation/CNN survey indicated that 90 percent of American adults believe the country is facing a mental health crisis attributable to illness and grief, loneliness and isolation, financial troubles and joblessness, among other consequences of a three-year pandemic.[16]

* * *

All of these mental health challenges did not emerge in a vacuum. They affected the behaviour of millions of people. Lockdowns increased our risk of substance abuse, drug overdoses, suicidal ideation, and even violence. The data compiled during the early parts of the pandemic was mixed and difficult to extrapolate, but as the pandemic settled into an endemic (when there are lower levels of infection localized in specific regions), we began seeing some longer-term impacts in these social and criminal indicators.

There is no doubt that substance abuse of alcohol and drugs increased over the past three years, but what often gets lost in this conversation is that we went into the pandemic with fairly high levels of substance use. A 2019 Statistics Canada report on drinking and drug use, the last before COVID hit, showed that 5.4 million Canadians were already exceeding guidelines for alcohol consumption, putting their long-term health at risk. This was especially pronounced among younger drinkers, 31 percent of whom were regularly exceeding guidelines. Forty-five percent of Canadians were using cannabis in 2019, compared to around 20 percent in 2012. What's more, those who smoked were smoking more often: 4.1 million Canadians reported using weed in the last thirty days compared to 1 million in 2017. And 4.7 million Canadians reported using cannabis in combination with other substances. Over three million Canadians were already at moderate risk of problematic use.[17]

Experts agree, based on research and clinical observation, that COVID-19 created a perfect storm of factors known to increase substance use and abuse. It's not complicated: people are more likely to make unhealthy decisions, including abusing alcohol and drugs, when they are stressed, lonely, and hopeless.

As we saw earlier, liquor sales in Canada jumped 17.5 percent in the very first lockdown. US data indicates that 13 percent of the population had turned to substances to cope as early as April 2020. A poll conducted for the Canadian Centre on Substance Abuse and Addiction in the first months of the pandemic found that 94 percent of Canadians were staying home more; of those, 18 percent said they were drinking more, mostly due to boredom and stress. Experts were already warning that the increases in consumption would "impact our health systems in the short and longer term, through increased hospitalizations due to alcohol-related illness, addiction, violence, and accidents."[18]

Over the longer course of the pandemic, Canadians over the age of fifteen reported a 24 percent increase in alcohol use (8 percent used less or the same) and a 34 percent increase in cannabis use (17 percent used less or the same).[19] The annual value of hard liquor sales across Canada stood at $5.5 billion in 2017/2018. It shot up in excess of 20 percent to 6.7 billion by 2021-2022 and the overall volume of alcohol sales was up about 12 percent for the same period.[20] In Ontario, there was a 22 percent increase in outpatient visits for severe alcohol use in the first fifteen months of the pandemic, offset somewhat by a 15 percent decline in emergency visits, yet the number of people needing to be hospitalized was up 6 percent.

That decline in emergency visits was at least partly a result of the lockdowns. Before the pandemic, it was more common for teens and people in their twenties to wind up in the hospital after drinking too much during a night out. Once COVID hit, the profile of the hospitalized drinker changed. It was more often people in their thirties. Their hospitalizations were up 22 percent from pre-pandemic levels.[21] The Canadian Institute for Health Information reported a total of 4,300 additional hospitalizations for alcohol-related conditions in the first sixteen months of the pandemic, not counting 8,000 more hospital stays for behavioural and mental disorders related to drinking.

Researchers at Massachusetts General Hospital used data from a national survey of US adults on their drinking habits and concluded excessive or "binge" drinking increased by 21 percent during the COVID-19 pandemic. They estimate that increased drinking has killed an additional 8,000 people from alcohol-related liver disease.[22]

Some might think that self-medicating with alcohol or cannabis helped people cope with the challenges of the pandemic. On the contrary, an article in BMC Psychiatry found that, overall, those who increased cannabis use during the pandemic were more prone to undergo meaningful perceived worsening of depression symptoms.[23]

Harder drugs presented harder problems with more serious consequences. Canada was already in the midst of an opioid crisis before the pandemic. A study released in the last month of 2019 found that 14,000 people had died of opioid overdoses and another 17,000 were hospitalized. This was when fentanyl, an extremely potent synthetic drug often mixed with heroin and other substances, was making its presence felt. The problem was extreme in British Columbia, which was reporting twenty-two deaths annually for every 100,000 residents. Its death toll from overdoses was 5,029 between 2016-2019. To put that in perspective, as of February 2023, B.C. had seen 5,106 people die of COVID-19.[24]

From March 2020 to September 2021, rates of emergency medical services in Ontario for suspected opioid overdoses jumped by 57 percent and fatal opioid overdoses increased by 60 percent. Fentanyl, sedatives, and stimulants were often identified as the drugs found in post-mortem toxicology reports. According to the Ontario Science Table: "Rural and Northern communities, people experiencing poverty or homelessness, people experiencing incarceration, and Black, Indigenous, People of Colour (BIPOC) communities have seen largest relative increases."[25]

British Columbia again was hardest hit. Its number of fatal overdoses almost doubled from 987 in 2019 to 1,774 in 2020 and jumped again to 2,306 in 2021, staying at that rate of more than six deaths a day in 2022. Most of the dead were male (79 percent) and located in or around Vancouver. One of the most marked changes in the composition of the victims during the pandemic is that older people were dying: 38 percent of the victims were over the age of fifty in 2022 compared to 30 percent in 2017.[26]

In Canada as a whole, the 2019 pre-pandemic rate of between 750 and 1,100 overdoses every three months leapt in 2020 and 2021 to between 1,700 and 2,200, with the peak occurring in the last quarter of 2021, about the time we were most fed up (and the Freedom Convoy was organized). In the first six months of 2022, 3,556 people fatally overdosed in Canada for a rate of nineteen per 100,000 people, almost level with British Columbia's alarming pre-pandemic levels. Almost all of these deaths (87 percent) occurred in Ontario, B.C., and Alberta; the vast majority of the victims were male (75 percent).

All told, Canada has experienced 34,455 opioid toxicity deaths since 2016, which is two-thirds our total number of COVID-19 deaths. While there is some suggestion that opioid-related deaths are falling in 2023, a range of scenarios modelled by the Public Health Agency of Canada suggests that, at best, we're still likely to see numbers elevated well above 2019 levels this year. In the worst-case scenario, we could remain at peak-pandemic levels for the foreseeable future.[27]

Terrible as those numbers are they remain well below American levels. The pandemic pushed the rate of overdoses per 100,000 people from 21.6 in 2019 to 28.3 in 2020.[28] Most states saw increases in opioid-related mortality along with ongoing concerns for those with substance use disorders. In 2021, America saw more than 100,000 deaths caused by opioids.[29]

Some psychologists monitoring this crisis believe the increase in overdoses may be due to substance misuse; that is, overdoses that occur when people do drugs alone and there is no one to call 911 or administer naloxone (opioid-reversal agent). Increased isolation during lockdowns presented a genuine risk for drug users, as disruptions in the drug supply chain resulted in more incidents of stronger or spiked drugs.[30]

* * *

One of the great fears in the early days of the pandemic was that the obvious distress people were under would push up the suicide rate, domestic violence rates, and crime rates. The data does not bear this out but, at the same time, there's not a lot to be cheerful about.

A review of twenty-one countries ranging from middle-income to high-income found no evidence of a significant increase in the risk of suicide death since the start of the pandemic.[31] This is consistent with a July 2022 Canadian study that found suicides decreased by 15 percent during the pandemic.

While the number of suicides did not increase, suicidal ideation did, indicating that many people were desperately struggling to keep themselves together. Several Canadian surveys conducted by Leger from March 2020 found the overall rate of those contemplating suicide was around 8 percent in January 2022.[32] That was up from 4.2 percent shortly after the start of the pandemic. The pre-pandemic level was 2.7 percent.[33] A statistically significant increase in prevalence was observed among those younger than age sixty-five, born in Canada, with lower levels of education, and living in Ontario or Western Canada.

Leger also found that people with histories of substance use disorders were increasingly likely to contemplate suicide seriously as the pandemic progressed. By June 2021, 22 percent were considering suicide, up from 13 percent in November 2020. By January 2022, the number had increased to over 30 percent (with men slightly over-represented compared to women).[34]

The immediate impact of COVID-19 on crime rates was mixed. A massive twenty-seven city, twenty-three country survey of criminal activity found that lockdowns resulted in declines in all manner of crime except homicide. With more people at home, there were fewer opportunities for residential burglary. With fewer people on the street, there was less street crime. With fewer young men out partying at night, there were fewer getting drunk and disorderly, driving drunk, and fighting.

However, only three cities, all in South America, showed statistically significant declines in the homicide rate. Two reasons may be that a substantial proportion of killings occur in the home and many more are associated with organized crime which was not disrupted by COVID to the same extent as other segments of society. As the lockdowns were relaxed, levels of criminal activity tended to return to the pre-pandemic norm.[35]

At the start of the pandemic, Canadians were worried about what might happen on their streets. A survey from March-April 2020 showed 40 percent of us were very or extremely concerned about the possibility of civil disorder. In fact, our experience was consistent with global patterns: overall crime levels decreased during the pandemic, especially in the first year. Our property crime rate was the lowest it had been since 1965. In 2021, some categories such as assault, sexual assault, robbery, and motor vehicle theft increased significantly over 2020. In fact, sexual assault crimes were up 18 percent in 2021, driving an increase in overall violent crime numbers to levels higher than those seen in 2019.

One outlier throughout the pandemic was hate crimes. Police reports showed a 37 percent increase in hate crimes in 2020 over 2019, climbing to the highest levels ever recorded in Canada. Black, Asian, and Indigenous populations were the primary targets. Given what we've already seen about anger, rage, and mental illness, it's perhaps not surprising that hate crimes spiked.

Another exception to the lower crime trend in Canada was the homicide rate. In the ten years before COVID-19, we had been averaging about 600 homicides a year, a number that crept up to about 670 a year for the period 2017-2019. In the first year of the pandemic, homicides jumped to 759 and in 2021 to 788. Both were Canadian records.[36] One hundred and fifty-four of the homicides in 2021 were committed by a family member compared to 145 in 2019.[37]

Early in the lockdowns, the United Nations was warning of a "shadow pandemic" of intimate partner violence. The *American Journal of Emergency Medicine* reported that domestic violence cases increased by 25 to 33 percent globally. Criminal justice data showed a smaller but still significant increase of 8 percent.[38]

In Canada, police reported 114,132 cases of intimate partner violence in 2021, up 4 percent from 2019. However, there was a large (22 percent) increase in sexual assault among intimate partners. And it may be that police reports don't accurately reflect what was happening in our homes. For long periods during the pandemic, calls to women's helplines were double the levels of pre-pandemic times. We know from experience that problems generally start long before they're reported. "Statistics tell us that domestic violence goes on long before someone actually picks up the phone to call the police," says Sgt. Julie Randall of the Ontario Provincial Police. "So, anecdotally, I can say that often our calls are lower than what's actually happening in the community."

Most of the domestic violence was directed at women, consistent with past experience, but an unusually high proportion of it was aimed at seniors. Not only were the elderly at greater risk of dying from infection but they were also subjected to much higher rates of violent attack often at the hands of loved ones. Family violence against seniors was up 8 percent in 2021 over 2020, and 14 percent higher than in 2019. Regrettably, family violence against seniors is up 37 percent since 2009.[39] Children were not immune to abuse and violence. Parents admitted to being tougher on their kids when are stressed.[40]

A whole other set of pandemic effects on crime statistics may just be materializing now. Emptying downtown cores have combined with higher levels of addiction, mental health problems and homelessness to the detriment of our larger cities. Alexandra Hryciw is chair of Edmonton's Downtown Recovery Coalition, which was founded last year in response to storefronts being smashed and pedestrians being accosted or assaulted in the city's core. "Edmonton is not an anomaly," she says. "Cities across North America are struggling with the impacts of the pandemic on their downtown cores. There's been a heightened safety issue that Edmonton's been addressing just in terms of houselessness and mental health and addictions."[41]

In Vancouver, stranger attacks increased dramatically by 35 percent in 2021-22 compared to 2019-2020. [42] Recently the TTC, Toronto's public transit system, has seen a sharp increase in violence, with an average of 2.4 offenses for every million times someone got onto a TTC vehicle in December 2022. This represented an increase from 1.85 per million in November 2022.[43] In March 2023, a young man was stabbed to death in one of the subway stations. [44]

As recently as September 2022, a group of researchers in British Columbia reconfirmed that most people with mental illness never become violent or commit criminal acts. There is no doubt, however, that the impact of mental health combined with changing types of recreational drug use and having more toxic illicit drug supplies in circulation contributes to unpredictable behaviour. Methamphetamine-induced psychosis has skyrocketed in emergency departments. There is a moderate but significant association between psychotic disorders and violence. Health-care professionals are now seeing higher rates of violence from people who were never seen to have acted violently in the past.[45]

* * *

Before we leave this part of our discussion, we need to look at what actually happened with vaccines since they became the focus of so much controversy, misinformation, and mental stress during the pandemic.

In Canada, approximately 97,000,000 vaccine doses had been administered as of February 2023. We were highly compliant when it came to getting our first vaccine dose and, as mentioned earlier, less so for subsequent doses and boosters.[46]

Over 95 percent of administered doses were mRNA vaccines made by Pfizer and Moderna and less than 5 percent were the traditional type of vaccine made by AstraZeneca.[47] It is the view of the vast majority of scientists and physicians that the mRNA vaccines have been literal lifesavers on a population-wide scale. Almost everyone who had the Pfizer or Moderna vaccines experienced them not only as highly effective but safe, with negligible side effects. As with all drugs, some complications did result in some people, but overall, these new mRNA vaccines were and continue to be scientific miracles.

Adverse events (side effects) were reported by approximately 55,000 Canadians. That's about 6 out of every 10,000 vaccinated. Of these, most were considered mild or non-serious, such as soreness at the site of injection or a slight fever (0.045 percent of all doses administered) and the rest were considered serious, including instances of anaphylaxis, a severe allergic reaction (0.011 percent of all doses administered).[48] This is a massive success story for any drug or vaccine.

Most of the side effects were found in the early use of the AstraZeneca and Janssen vaccines, which were quickly dropped once the mRNA vaccines became more widely available. [49]As noted earlier, the AstraZeneca vaccine was given first to those considered most at risk, primarily seniors. In Canada, it was also given initially to those over age fifty-five. Approximately three months after this vaccine was distributed, the European Medicines Agency, similar to the Federal Drug Administration in the United States, sent out the following warning:

> EMA is reminding health-care professionals and people receiving the vaccine to remain aware of the possibility of very rare cases of blood clots combined with low levels of blood platelets occurring within 2 weeks of vaccination. So far, most of the cases reported have occurred in women under 60 years of age within 2 weeks of vaccination. Based on the currently available evidence, specific risk factors have not been confirmed.[50]

Scientists would later discover that the AstraZeneca vaccine created an adverse immune response, resulting in a combination of blood clots and low blood platelets. Such a condition has been observed in patients treated with heparin, which they call HIT or heparin-induced thrombocytopenia.[51]

Because this vaccine was targeting the original Wuhan virus, it was largely ineffective for the Delta strain of the second wave. Those who received AZ essentially got a placebo and had to wait far longer for an effective second mRNA shot, which would be their booster many months later than most of the population had completed their primary series of two mRNA vaccines.

The rate of adverse event reports was highest among the forty to forty-nine-year age group (82.4 reports per 100,000 doses administered), followed by those in the thirty to thirty-nine-year age group (70.2 reports per 100,000 doses administered).[52]

Overall, most adverse event reports were from females (72.7 percent). The reporting rate for females was 75.8 reports per 100,000 doses administered, compared to 30.6 per 100,000 doses administered for males. However, within the youngest age groups (under eighteen years of age) the reporting rate is either similar in males and females, or slightly higher in males.[53]

I would never have thought that a pandemic crisis could have resulted in such extraordinary volumes of false information. The AI algorithms are partly to blame, but their content was created by real people. Throughout the pandemic, health-care professionals were not only fighting COVID-19 but scientific and medical misinformation spread far and wide by the malicious and misinformed. There is no doubt that some of this led to unnecessary sickness and death because of people not taking vaccines or opting for alternative and ineffective treatments such as the equine drug Ivermectin.[54]

A study commissioned by The Council of Canadian Academies found misinformation led to the belief that COVID-19 was fake or that its danger was exaggerated, resulting in more vaccine hesitancy: 2.35 million people decided to delay or refuse the vaccine in the early waves of the pandemic when the more deadly and serious strains were circulating. [55] The council estimates that more than 2,800 Canadians died unnecessarily and that the health-care system suffered at least $300 million in unnecessary hospital and ICU visits.

The true costs to the health-care system are likely far higher, given that the model did not include the cost of those who did not enter the hospital but nevertheless required physician care. Nor did it capture ripple effects across society, including the opportunities for the spread of new variants and the strains they placed on Canada's health-care system, and a slowed economic recovery.

The council called the consequences of the misinformation sad and unfortunate. That's an understatement. Most health-care professionals, including myself, viewed the misinformation as ignorant and stupid. It was the last thing we needed while fighting to care for the lives of everyone, regardless of their personal beliefs.

and the strains they placed on Canada's health-care system, and slowed economic recovery.

The control called the consequences of the misinformation sad and unfortunate. That's an understatement. Most health-care professionals, including myself, viewed the misinformation as ignorant and stupid. It was the last thing we needed while fighting to care for the lives of everyone regardless of their personal beliefs.

CHAPTER FOUR

LIVING IN A POST-TRAUMATIC SOCIETY

Whether or not you were infected, you are a survivor of COVID-19. It was virtually impossible not to be touched in one way or another by the whole ordeal. Our lives were turned upside down. The cumulative trauma of the pandemic is something that weighs heavily on my mind. On a societal level, we have bigger problems than we've acknowledged.

Let's start with the microtrauma. These is just as it sounds: a small version of trauma, which is defined as lasting emotional response to living through a distressing event. Microtraumas are small enough that you might not recognize them as traumatic when they happen and, individually, they likely have a minor impact on how we feel. But enough of them spread over time can have a detrimental effect on your well-being, just as enough of them spread over an entire population can be damaging to society.

Like regular trauma, microtrauma affects us by activating our stress response systems, which in turn determine how we feel and act, resulting in physical and social consequences. Some of these consequences are good, leading to kindness and altruistic acts. Others are not so good, leading to angry outbursts and violent acts. They can program assumptions into our brains, leading us to respond reflexively to circumstances, perhaps by lashing out, withdrawing from the world, over-eating or drinking too much.

Here's a brief reminder of some of the pandemic's microtraumatic events and jarring realities that we've all dealt with over the last three years:

63

discovering that a lethal virus was circulating the world and, eventually, in our workplaces, communities, and perhaps our homes; confusion about viral transmission (first focusing on air droplets and cleaning surfaces, only to discover later it was primarily airborne); conflicting advice and changing recommendations around masking; global shortages of personal protective equipment; the lack of proven drugs or vaccines for the first year of the pandemic; a sudden shift to working and schooling from home; regional and international border shutdowns; conflicting advice and rampant misinformation about vaccines and their potential risks versus benefits; social isolation; the constant threat of new variants and other viruses arriving; an economic crash, a stock market meltdown, rampant inflation, and other economic dislocation.

One or two of these microtraumas are probably manageable for most people. Each of us might be better positioned to cope with some challenges than others. The effect of a specific event is different from person to person depending on individual circumstances and individual experiences associated with the microtrauma; similar to how a Canadian city can generally manage well with a major snowstorm while a minor snowfall in Dallas can cause chaos. But *cumulatively* these things can affect us in a manner similar to major trauma, leading to negative responses detrimental to ourselves and those around us. In other words, a string of microtraumas can lead to a medical condition known as post-traumatic stress disorder (PTSD).

The potential for microtrauma was high almost everywhere you looked during the pandemic. Think about what's happened in your own family and what you've heard about other people's families. There were serious disagreements about the severity of COVID-19 and what accommodations needed to be made for it. There were arguments over how seriously to take lockdowns, restrictions on group activities, and travel bans. There were fights over the new demands of child-care and on-line schooling and work-from-home, as one would expect when the basic social structures of society changed overnight. Individuals were suddenly thrust into caregiving roles with sick spouses or elderly parents who were having difficulty coping on their own. The question of whether or not vaccines were advisable or necessary ripped some families and friendships apart. Even loving families found it difficult to spend a lot of time cooped up together over the long haul. Again, most people would have been capable of dealing with one or two of these things, but a bunch of them in succession amounted to trauma.

Of course, many people also suffered full-scale trauma during the pandemic. They saw their businesses ruined, or were victims of intimate partner violence, or watched loved ones hospitalized or taken by COVID-19. While, again, each person has a unique response to their specific loss or losses, there can be no doubt that many of us will endure lasting effects from trauma and loss.

We often equate the term post-traumatic stress disorder with war veterans who have been involved in an overseas deployment or first responders who witness the effects of a crime, such as a mass shooting. In fact, PTSD is a disorder that can develop in anyone who has experienced a shocking, scary, or dangerous event. Feeling fear during or after a traumatic situation triggers a fight-or-flight response caused by the secretion of cortisol hormone, which in turn triggers the secretion of adrenalin. This chemical causes our heart rate and blood pressure to rise. We feel more "ready to go" and are more prepared to protect ourselves and others from harm. Most people recover from these transient symptoms. However, those who continue to experience fear, anxiety, and depression, even without any dangerous triggers, may be diagnosed with PTSD.[1]

Perhaps the best illustration I can offer of how PTSD works is to share my own experience. I mentioned earlier my encounter with the SARS epidemic of 2003. It was a frightening time, not least because I was on the front lines and had a young child whose safety I was particularly worried about. Both of his parents, uncle, and grandfather were all directly involved in the fight against SARS in Toronto.

When COVID-19 emerged early in 2020, I was glued to the news. For the sake of my patients, I had to stay on top of worldwide health and medical news. That's not usually too difficult or time-consuming, but the COVID updates were fast and furious. The flood of statistics, images, and stories that emerged in those early weeks was spectacular and overwhelming. There were exponential rates of infections and death around the world. Hospital staffs were working with inadequate PPE, begging and crying for masks, gloves, and gowns. Emails from University Health Network, our largest hospital system in Canada, outlined how all staff could store, reuse, and re-sanitize their daily rations of masks. Nurses posted on social media to show others how to make masks from T-shirts and gowns from garbage bags. Field hospitals were constructed in my community teaching hospital.

One night in mid-March, after an anxious week getting my son safely home from college, I lost it. I was watching an evening newscast of yet another horrible day for hospital doctors and nurses trying to do their best work with the equipment (or lack thereof) on hand. I began to cry.

My son said: "What's wrong with you, Mom? You don't need to cry. It's not you and not your patients."

That sent me on a tirade. Tears streaming down my face, I said something like, "But it could be me! It could be my clinic patients or my nursing home patients! It could have been you! While you are safely home playing video games and eating home-cooked meals and enjoying clean laundry, your dad's and mom's friends are risking their lives every day to deal with stupid people who refuse to listen to science-based health advice to stay away from each other and simply wear a mask! They could die and leave their kids without parents."

The flood of my current fears, combined with the anxiety I experienced during SARS, boiled over. I proceeded to tell him what we'd had to do in 2003 to keep him safe. My meltdown probably lasted fifteen minutes. I was sobbing and screaming at him. He has never again asked me, "What's wrong?" Because everything was *really* wrong.

All of which is to say that we've each incurred bills in this pandemic that will come due in the future. There will be new pain points, new vulnerabilities, heightened sensitivities, and all manner of delayed reactions to what we endured, few of them positive. We are now living in a post-traumatic society.

* * *

We might think the pandemic has blown over and things are back to normal, but it may only take one incident, one memory, one word, to tip us over the edge again. Human beings don't always react immediately to trauma and loss, as Elisabeth Kübler-Ross famously demonstrated with her five stages of grief. Some of us will deny as long as possible that we've been seriously injured by what happened. Some will be stuck for a long time in anger, maybe acting out on Twitter or joining a Freedom Convoy. The journey continues on through bargaining, which can take the form of numbing themselves through substance abuse, to depression and, finally, acceptance. It can take many years and still leave one susceptible to post-traumatic reactions.

I especially worry about the health-care professionals who bore the brunt of the pandemic's first wave and, really, every subsequent wave. They are trained to manage specific situations. Physicians know how to stop bleeding from an injury and methodically control the sources of bleeding. Their training and their experience help them dampen the risk that a potential event becomes materially traumatic. But as we all know, health-care workers are not immune to trauma despite their training, particularly if an event is gruesome and unpredictable.

No amount of training can prepare you for the challenge of confronting a mysterious and deadly virus without sufficient PPE, or effective medications, or seeing *hundreds* of people die in ICU and hospital wards. Hospital staff endured eighteen months of repeated exposure to sick COVID-19 patients before vaccines became widely available and administered. Overburdened and unrested, they were asked to do things that no one was trained to do in any industrialized country. One-time use of proper PPE is an infection-control basic. It is drilled into every health-care worker to never compromise on this point. As mentioned above, health workers suddenly had no choice. They did the best they could under the circumstances while realizing that they could be infecting each other and killing the next patient while reusing protective equipment or going without any at all.[2]

Those were only the beginning of the unreasonable demands. Physicians were asked to triage who would get ventilators, beds, monoclonal antibody treatments, and, in some countries (mercifully, not Canada) even oxygen. This was and continues to be a significant psychological burden for every health-care worker who endured it.

There are undoubtedly many cases of PTSD among health-care professionals. All through the pandemic, they faced long working hours, loneliness, inadequate rest and self-care, feelings of helplessness, and occasional violence and threats from angry patients and family, not to mention pandemic deniers. Then, in late 2022, they were subjected to the "tripledemic" of COVID, influenza, and RSV (respiratory syncytial virus). Family time and the support of loved ones, a common de-stressor for these workers, were often denied them because of the need to stay away from loved ones to prevent the spread of infection. With next to nothing in the way of ongoing PTSD support at work and ongoing high volumes of patient care, many of them resigned from burnout. This has led to even greater staffing issues and more work for those who remain on the job.

A third of the UK's health-care workers reported moderate to severe levels of anxiety and depression; the number of people who reported "very high" symptoms quadrupled. In the view of some researchers, the most severe levels of psychiatric symptoms would have been "controllable" had the health-care system been better prepared.[3]

Despite taking what precautions they could, many health-care workers did get sick while caring for patients in hospitals and clinics. A February 2023 study from the United Kingdom looked at approximately 500 patients from the first (original strain) and second wave (Delta strain) of COVID-19 and found that these patients were far more likely to have Long COVID. One-third of them were health-care workers. Sixty-two percent had some form of organ impairment six months after their initial diagnosis. Fifty-nine percent had a single organ impairment and 30 percent of them had multi-organ impairment with persistent Long COVID symptoms twelve months after initial diagnosis.[4]

In 2022, the Registered Practical Nurses' Association of Ontario conducted a survey of its members in which six in ten reported that their mental health had deteriorated in the pandemic and an astonishing 47 percent were considering leaving nursing, up from 24 percent at the end of the first year of COVID (Ontario went into the pandemic with a shortfall of 22,000 registered nurses on a per capita basis compared to the rest of Canada).[5]

Amid all of the pandemic's pain and suffering, there were some positive developments in the health-care world. As in-person medical appointments virtually disappeared, virtual visits became a lifeline to continuity of care as lockdowns began to roll out throughout the world. Although telemedicine has been available for decades in Canada to support hard-to-reach rural and northern communities, virtual care became front and centre in 2020. This is incredibly valuable in a world where, according to Angus Reid, more than 6,000,000 Canadian adults don't have access to a family doctor.[6] Virtual care is a valuable asset in dealing with this crisis.

It *is* a crisis, our doctor shortage, and the pandemic made it worse. A 2022 study led by Unity Health Toronto and published in *Annals of Family Medicine* determined that family doctors in Ontario were leaving the profession at double the rate they had in the years before the pandemic. Said Dr. Tara Kiran, lead author of the report, "We hypothesize that what probably happened is the pandemic and those stresses and challenges and worries probably accelerated their retirement plans." Canada needs to train or hire 30,000 more physicians by 2028 to match the average number of doctors per capita among OECD peers.

* * *

The loss of health-care professionals is yet another bill society will have to pay for the pandemic in the years ahead. It would require another book to inventory them all, but here are a few more by way of example.

Not all front-line workers were in health care. There were many others who were required to show up for work in extremely difficult circumstances. Many of them worked in retail and food services: grocery stores, pharmacies, food processing plants, warehouses, and other facilities had to keep operating, as did trucking firms and delivery services. These are the people who packaged our hand sanitizer shipments and bagged our groceries and provided all kinds of other services so that the rest of us could survive the ordeal. Those taking care of our most vulnerable— our elderly, new immigrants, refugees, the unhoused, the addicted, the mentally ill—also had to remain at their posts.

We called them essential workers and yet gave them little in the way of additional support. Their jobs often paid poorly and lacked security. They often risked greater exposure to the virus than those who could remain at home in front of their computers. Many were left feeling taken for granted. The pandemic exacerbated ugly inequalities and social divisions in our society. We can expect repercussions in our politics in the years ahead.

Children who contracted COVID-19 tended to fare well. Compared with other age groups, the overall risk of death from COVID-19 was substantially lower for them (it was the underlying cause of 2 percent of deaths in children and young people).[7] The pandemic's true impact on children will come in the form of delayed development, the consequences of which may play out throughout their lifetimes.

Academic, emotional, and social skill development was put on hold for our kids as they languished at home for the better part of two years: 1.6 billion students in 194 countries were impacted by school closures.[8] The digital divide was acutely revealed. According to UNICEF, only one-third of the world's school-age children have Internet access at home.[9] Three in ten Canadian families could not access the Internet to attend online classes at home. Many of these children used public Wi-Fi to complete assignments. It has been estimated that globally students experienced learning loss of about 35 percent during each of the past two years as in-person learning was repeatedly interrupted, and that's assuming students were able to access their lessons.[10]

Many schools are now experiencing an explosion of anxiety disorders among teenagers. It is notable that, regardless of age, educators observed children struggling to reintegrate into classrooms; they needed to relearn basic socialization skills.[11] In 2019, 73 percent of those aged twelve to seventeen described their mental health as very good or excellent, but by 2022 that number had declined to 61 percent. Eating disorder rates rose during the pandemic, especially among girls, with more of them being admitted for non-suicidal self-harm and suicide presentations than boys.[12]

The World Health Organization ominously predicts that mental health disorders will be the world's leading cause of disability by 2030: "The consequences of failing to address adolescent mental health conditions extend to adulthood, impairing both physical and mental health and limiting opportunities to lead fulfilling lives as adults."[13] This should give us pause regarding the damage done to our youths.

There is also good reason to be concerned about the welfare of our seniors in the years ahead. The Commonwealth Fund survey of more than 18,000 adults age sixty-five and older in eleven high-income countries found COVID-19 significantly affected the economic security of older adults as well as their access to health care and supportive services for chronic conditions. With reduced social services and less social contact, in addition to low fixed incomes, many seniors had insufficiently nutritious diets and were cut off from supportive services, which impacted their ability to thrive during the pandemic.

North America, in particular, failed its seniors. Older Americans were four to six times more likely to have lost their job or used up all or most of their savings than seniors living in Germany, Switzerland, the Netherlands, Norway, and Sweden.[14] Compared to their counterparts in other countries, they were most likely to report that they did not receive needed help because supportive services became very limited or were cancelled during the pandemic.[15] One-third of Canadians reported pandemic-related disruptions in their care for chronic conditions. By contrast, German seniors reported that only 11 percent of their medical appointments were cancelled or postponed.[16]

The disruption of work is another thing that will take years to work out. Adria Horn, a McKinsey partner and a former lieutenant colonel in the US Army Reserve, served five tours of duty overseas between 2003 and 2010. In January 2021, she wrote an article for *McKinsey Quarterly* titled "A Military Veteran Knows Why Your Employees are Leaving."[17] It drew parallels between the struggles soldiers face returning home after deployment and those faced by employees trying to create a path forward and find a new normal at work during and after the pandemic. A chaplain once told her and her fellow returning veterans during a reintegration seminar that "things would feel different, that even though you're happy to be back, you'll feel like you don't fit in, that your house and your routine will feel strange, that your family won't understand you, and you won't understand them."

Workers, in a sense, were redeployed during the pandemic to a basement or spare bedroom at home. With the pandemic's passing, they are being redeployed again, sometimes to the office and sometimes to hybrid work. Some chief human resources officers I've spoken with admit this is a "social experiment."

It might have been expected that employees would have resisted a return to the office. In the first redeployment of early 2020, everyone was rolling with the punches for the common good. That feeling has long since worn off. Almost 60 percent of workers now say they can do their jobs from home and 60 percent of this group work from home all or most of the time.[18] People have developed new pandemic workstyles and living arrangements—many have moved out of downtown cores to more affordable and congenial environments. The lack of a commute has saved some families valuable time as well as money. The ordeal of COVID-19 prompted many people to adjust their priorities and reconsider what they want out of work, one of the reasons the number of people leaving and changing jobs is high.[19]

At the same time, business leaders are struggling to manage their teams without a full-time office presence. A number of high-profile companies such as Apple have asked employees to return. CEO Tim Cook insists that in-person collaboration is essential for his company. Royal Bank of Canada CEO David McKay struck a similar tone, saying "Technology can't replicate the energy, spontaneity, big ideas or true sense of belonging that comes from working together in person. Mentorship and skills development, critical parts of the bank's culture, are challenging when done through video screens." Both of these companies have met fierce resistance.[20] Admits McKay: "It's a difficult needle to move."[21]

There is good evidence that the new models of remote and hybrid work are here to stay.[22] So long as wages stay high and unemployment rates remain low,[23] there are no incentives to nudge employees to return to their workplaces full time. In my world of corporate wellness, I've been encouraging senior leadership to be selective in deciding which teams would benefit from in-person collaboration and ensure that in-office time is well spent on in-person collaboration and not virtual meetings done in office cubicles. Also, they need to prepare their employees for reintegration into the office. Otherwise, we'll be hearing a lot more about the "great resignation" and "quiet quitting." Deployment burnout and PTSD are real.

Of course, not everyone has a choice about leaving a job or whether or not to work. Many lost their positions, saw their hours reduced, or couldn't find employment. Even with massive government support programs, millions suffered financial setbacks. The loss of income was highest amongst women, who were disproportionately employed in sectors vulnerable to lockdowns; youth, the self-employed, and casual workers with lower levels of formal education were also hurt.[24] That the damage was concentrated among disadvantaged populations will increase income inequality in Canada and around the world, as if that problem weren't troubling enough before the pandemic.

The economic dimensions of the pandemic are far too broad to treat fully in this book. Suffice it to say that we are all living with the effects of high levels of government debt compounded by high consumer demand, rampant inflation, and high-interest rates. As noted in The Organization for Economic Cooperation and Development (OECD) economic outlook at the end of 2022: "Growth has lost momentum, high inflation has broadened out across countries and products and is proving persistent. Risks are skewed to the downside. Energy supply shortages could push prices higher. Interest rate increases are necessary to curb inflation and heighten financial vulnerabilities. Russia's war in Ukraine is increasing the risks of debt distress in low-income countries and food insecurity."[25]

That last point regarding food insecurity deserves additional attention. "Food security," according to a definition supplied by the 1996 World Food Summit, "is achieved when all people, at all times, have physical and economic access to sufficient, safe, and nutritious food to meet their dietary needs and food preferences for an active and healthy life."[26]

The pandemic put into sharp focus the vulnerability of our food system, particularly how we are organized to grow, harvest, pack, process, and transport food to the consumer. All of us experienced temporary shortages of certain food items due to border shutdowns and the weaknesses exposed in the pre-pandemic just-in-time inventory practice.

Cost inflation was seen across all food categories and placed additional unwelcome burdens on individuals and families with lower incomes. After a modest increase of 2.2 percent in 2021, reports Statistics Canada, prices in grocery stores rose 9.8 percent in 2022, the fastest pace since 1981.[27] According to Canada's Food Price Report 2023, a Canadian family of four will spend approximately $16,288 per year on food, a jump of $1,065 compared to 2022.[28]

We do not have the food security we've always thought we have. If we want to ensure reliable access to nutritious food, especially for our most vulnerable populations, we'll need to make major adjustments to our financial, inventory, and distribution systems in the years ahead.

If you live in an urban area and have walked around your downtown core recently, I don't need to tell you how much things have changed since COVID-19 emerged. Living in Toronto, I've seen our city's business core hollowed out. Many small businesses that used to support thousands of daily commuting workers with everything from meals, haircuts, and dry cleaning could not sustain their storefronts and have closed. Most major cities have experienced something similar. The National Association of Industrial and Office Properties predicts that office absorption will slow in 2023 due to economic uncertainty. Canada's downtown office vacancy rate reached 19 percent in March 2023, as cities such as Toronto and Vancouver shift to hybrid work. This level of vacancy is almost double the 10.8 percent in downtown markets before the start of the pandemic, according to Altus Group—the highest rate of vacancy since 2003.[29]

What will become of our downtowns is yet another problem we'll have to solve in the years ahead—another pandemic bill that will at some point come due. There are so many of them. That's what it means to live in a post-traumatic society.

CHAPTER FIVE

WHAT NEEDS TO BE DONE

Given all that's happened in the last three years, including the millions of people who were sick and the more than fifty thousand Canadians who died, our governments have been shockingly reluctant to review their performance, ask what they could have done better, and set us up for a greater degree of success when the next pandemic hits.

What would such a review look like? Something along the lines of what *The Lancet*, a medical journal, did on a global level, with the results published late last year. A year into the pandemic, *The Lancet* established a COVID-19 commission to develop recommendations on how best to suppress the virus, address the humanitarian, economic, and financial crises it produced, and "rebuild for an inclusive, fair, and sustainable world." Twenty-eight experts from all over the world met regularly starting in 2020 and oversaw specific task forces which drew in another 173 experts.

Here's what the commission determined:

> As of May 31, 2022, there were 6.9 million reported deaths and 17.2 million estimated deaths from COVID-19, as reported by the Institute for Health Metrics and Evaluation. This staggering death toll is both a profound tragedy and a massive global failure at multiple levels. Too many governments have failed to adhere to basic norms of institutional rationality and transparency, too many people—often

influenced by misinformation—have disrespected and protested against basic public health precautions, and the world's major powers have failed to collaborate to control the pandemic.

The multiple failures of international cooperation include (1) the lack of timely notification of the initial outbreak of COVID-19; (2) costly delays in acknowledging the crucial airborne exposure pathway of SARS-CoV-2, the virus that causes COVID-19, and in implementing appropriate measures at national and global levels to slow the spread of the virus; (3) the lack of coordination among countries regarding suppression strategies; (4) the failure of governments to examine evidence and adopt best practices for controlling the pandemic and managing economic and social spillovers from other countries; (5) the shortfall of global funding for low-income and middle-income countries (LMICs), as classified by the World Bank; (6) the failure to ensure adequate global supplies and equitable distribution of key commodities—including protective gear, diagnostics, medicines, medical devices, and vaccines—especially for LMICs; (7) the lack of timely, accurate, and systematic data on infections, deaths, viral variants, health system responses, and indirect health consequences; (8) the poor enforcement of appropriate levels of biosafety regulations in the lead-up to the pandemic, raising the possibility of a laboratory-related outbreak; (9) the failure to combat systematic disinformation; and (10) the lack of global and national safety nets to protect populations experiencing vulnerability.

It's quite an indictment. Perhaps that's why our governments don't want to put themselves through a similar exercise and lay bare the role they played in a "massive global failure"—how they were too slow and cautious in their response to the virus, how they failed the millions who got sick and the most vulnerable groups in our society, resulting in tens of thousands of preventable deaths.

But, again, we owe it to the dead, the sick, the traumatized, the dislocated, and the ruined. We owe it to ourselves to fully understand what happened, to acknowledge our failures and what we could have done better, and to make sure we don't repeat our mistakes in the future.

One unmistakable outcome of the pandemic was an erosion of trust in governments and institutions and public health. We should be worried about that. If these bodies can't be accepted as trusted and respected sources of apolitical truth and genuine guidance on how to safeguard our health and well-being, nothing will change. We might have demonstrated an ability to pull together and create life-saving vaccines in record time, but these advances, together with improvements in monitoring and early detection of viruses, will be useless. They will fall on deaf ears, with deadly consequences. You don't rebuild public trust by sweeping a pandemic under the carpet.

I urge our federal government to look in the mirror. Only its senior personnel know if we are better ready for the next pandemic than we were three years ago. If we're not, and I don't see much reason to think we are, we certainly can't blame it on a lack of health-care spending. At $331 billion in 2022, or $8,563 per Canadian, our public health funding is near the highest it has ever been (but for the pandemic peak). On a per capita basis, we spend more than many other developed countries,[1] but this does not necessarily mean better wait times and health outcomes.[2] We have a bad habit of comparing ourselves only the US and thinking that because we've escaped some of the failures and excesses of their system, ours is just fine. It isn't.

The Commonwealth Fund undertook a health-care system performance ranking for eleven major countries: Australia, Canada, France, Germany, the Netherlands, New Zealand, Norway, Sweden, Switzerland, the UK and US. The good news is we ranked better than the US. The bad news is that the US placed eleventh. We were tenth, performing abysmally on health-care outcomes (recovery and survival rates), equity, and access to care, and not much better on administrative efficiency.

That is not good enough. Not even close.

There's enough money in the system. The problem is that it's spent in a sub-optimal manner. Wrote Armine Yalnizyan, a senior economist at the Canadian Centre for Policy Alternatives: "There are a few old adages that we should apply to health budgeting decisions: A stitch in time saves nine. An ounce of prevention is worth a pound of cure. Let's not be penny-wise and pound foolish. Our goal should be to prevent the preventable and save health-care costs because we are improving health."[3]

We cannot keep throwing more money at disease care. We must invest more in primary prevention with better education and early detection of chronic health conditions. With the right information and incentives, people are capable of proactively managing their health. We need a health-care system reconfigured to help them do so. In this regard, our system is too much like its American counterpart, which in 2020 dedicated a measly 3 percent of its $3.6 trillion in health spending toward public health and prevention.[4] That's how you end up with the world's worst obesity problem.

The Government of Canada announced in 2022 that it was investing $10 million through the Canadian Institutes of Health Research and the Public Health Agency of Canada to increase public health research capacity in Canada. This includes $8 million for seven new applied public health chairs and $2 million for new research to address population and public health priorities. Again, it's nowhere near good enough.[5]

The scientific community, too, has more work to do. We need to understand why we've seen so many of these viruses emerge over the last thirty or forty years, starting with AIDS. Is our way of life becoming unsustainable, even dangerous?

As our populations expand, we are dwelling closer and closer to wildlife, requiring greater deforestation and urbanization, which are both contributing to and exacerbated by climate change. Our food supply relies on factory farming, in which hundreds of thousands of animals, such as chickens and pigs, are crammed together, becoming enormous potential petri dishes for spreading infection. These are among the factors that have many scientists concluding that the next pandemic is a 'when', not an 'if'. Effective preparation can't be achieved without multilateral cooperation, perhaps located at the global headquarters of a more effective and credible World Health Organization. We cannot leave it to local governments to manage viruses that know no borders.

Whether or not all this work will get done remains to be seen. We're certainly not off to a running start. In the meantime, it falls to all of us to do what we can to improve our own physical health and well-being. COVID-19 was a wake-up call for all who have been unhealthy. We risk self-harm if we don't manage our personal risk factors for developing chronic health issues such as cardiovascular disease, diabetes, cancer, and reduced immunity.

Let me be your doctor for a moment. Here's how you can help yourself do better.

A 2017 Canadian public health report found that 64 percent of Canadians over the age of eighteen are overweight. So lose it. If you're carrying around more pounds than you need, you are at risk of developing high blood pressure, high blood sugar, unhealthy cholesterol levels, diabetes, and cardiovascular disease, among much else. Change your diet. Move more. Get a good night's sleep.

Too many of us are stressed out and sleep deprived. That can lead to a lack of energy and motivation, poor concentration, lower levels of satisfaction, a sense of failure and self-doubt, and detachment. It can leave us anxious, headachy, irritable, and angry. Again, eat well, get a good night's sleep, and lay off the drugs and alcohol.

Managing your hormones becomes increasingly important as you age. Talk to your doctor about your estrogen, testosterone, and DHEA. These affect your weight, your bone loss, your ability to sleep, your strength, your libido, your mental health, your brain function, and your susceptibility to disease.

Finally, practice self care. As mentioned above, we have a "sick-care" system, not a "health-care" system. Until that changes, it's up to you to keep an eye on yourself and modify your behaviour to support your overall health and well-being. Pay attention to how you feel physically, emotionally, and spiritually and what makes you feel that way. Keep in shape and build your heart and lung capacity. Get your check-ups and scans. If medicines are prescribed for you, take them (20 to 30 percent of new prescriptions are never filled and half the time the medication is not taken).[6] Set healthy goals for yourself and be determined to sustain a healthy lifestyle. There will always be setbacks, but so long as you keep pursuing your long-term health goals, you are doing well.

World Health Organization data shows that 80 percent of cardiovascular diseases, diabetes, and cancer are preventable. These health conditions are some of the top reasons people ended up in the hospital or ICU once they got infected with COVID-19 and before vaccines became available. If you take better care of yourself, you'll be more resilient in the face of illnesses of the body and mind, including future epidemics and pandemics.

If nothing else, the last three years proved that we are not okay, but if we understand what we've been through and how to respond properly, we can all live longer, healthier, and disease-free lives.

RESPONSE TO SUTHERLAND QUARTERLY ISSUE 2, 2023

By Andrew Lawton

In the final week of the Public Order Emergency Commission's hearings last fall, Prime Minister Justin Trudeau needed to convince commissioner Paul Rouleau that he and his cabinet were justified in invoking the Emergencies Act to end the Freedom Convoy protests. Built into the Emergencies Act is a multi-point legal test for its invocation, which requires a "threat to the security of Canada."

As for what constitutes a "threat to the security of Canada," the Emergencies Act refers to a definition in the Canadian Security Intelligence Service Act. Much of the Rouleau Commission's work was reduced to painfully specific debate over one clause of one section of the CSIS Act. There was so much nitpicking over the interpretation of a "threat to the security of Canada," which CSIS itself advised the government did not exist during the Freedom Convoy, that I was convinced the federal government had lost its case. It seemed to me that if the question was so closely fought, if the situation was so delicately on the line that a slight breeze could have pushed it in either way, then surely so drastic a measure as Emergencies Act was unnecessary.

My instinct was wrong. Trudeau managed a legal win, which he has since framed as a moral victory.

Given that the narrow legal debate sucked much of the oxygen out of the Rouleau Commission. I was glad that it barely registered in Paul Wells' account of the hearings in *An Emergency in Ottawa*.

As he wrote, "The Rouleau Commission was about a drama, but it wasn't drama." That it wasn't drama is meaningful. As someone sympathetic (though not unquestioningly so) of the convoy, I admit I went into the hearings with a bit of trepidation. I had defended the convoy as a peaceful protest whose bad actors were not only very few in number but, crucially, had been denounced by those with moral sway over the protest.

Was I certain?

No.

Could there have been a darker element? Would the government hinge its case on a previously-undisclosed bombshell exposing the protest as far from peaceful? It wasn't implausible.

Two days after the Emergencies Act was invoked, Public Safety Minister Marco Mendicino held a press conference in which he proclaimed the existence of a "far-right, extreme organization with leaders who are in Ottawa" with plans to "overthrow the existing government." After a few pointed questions from reporters, he walked that statement back to concern over disturbing rhetoric on social media. But maybe he knew something.

The Public Order Emergency Commission found no evidence of a violent conspiracy, or the presence of weapons, or a plot to overthrow the government, save for the widely ridiculed (including by convoy supporters) "memorandum of understanding" circulated by one participant before and during the protest.

Without such evidence, it's difficult to see a threat to the security of the nation, yet that does not seem to bother those who supported (or at least made peace with) use of the Emergencies Act. As far as they're concerned, the convoy was a menace, the act was invoked, the convoy was dismantled. End justifies means, never mind the implications for political protest in Canada.

What I hoped might come of the commission was something resembling a cross-partisan agreement on the limits of protest, a standard that doesn't come down to whether or not we align with the cause being advocated.

Many who supported the Freedom Convoy had no patience for the 2020 anti-pipeline rail blockades, ostensibly in support of Wet'suwet'en First Nation. The hypocrisy ran the other way, too. Many who cheered the long-running Wet'suwet'en protest were delighted that Trudeau used the Emergencies Act to clear out the convoy.

NDP leader Jagmeet Singh, who supported the use of the Emergencies Act, was oddly transparent about his ideological litmus test for the right to protest: "Indigenous land defenders, climate change activists, workers fighting for fairness, and any Canadian using their voice to peacefully demand justice should never be subject to the Emergencies Act," he said on February 17, 2022.

We remain far from an agreement around protest rights.

While I could quibble with Wells on a few of his takeaways and his liberal use of the word "occupation" to describe the protest, his account is fair and insightful. It dutifully unpacks the intergovernmental and multijurisdictional intrigue that hampered the police response to the convoy (far more than the absence of emergency powers).

Where I diverge from Wells is on his assertion that the social divisions of the pandemic are largely over: "By the time everyone sat down for six weeks of testimony, the deep social fracture that had given rise to the Freedom Convoy had gone dormant again."

There are Covid alarmists and anti-restriction absolutists who have refused to move on from the pandemic era, which is why freedom rallies and calls for re-upping mask mandates persist, albeit in far smaller numbers than previously.

Politicians still see opportunities to score points. In April 2023, fourteen months after the fact, the British Columbia legislature voted almost unanimously to "denounce the Freedom Convoy protests and affirm that public health orders, including vaccine requirements, have been an essential tool in BC's response to the COVID-19 pandemic." The legislature's lone Conservative member voted against.

It would be a mistake to downplay how much harm and social division resulted from the pandemic cocktail of lockdowns, restrictions, and mandates. Justin Trudeau might have called for "healing as a nation" in the days after police dispersed the convoy. But that rang false for protesters and their supporters. It was less than a month earlier that he'd branded them a "fringe minority" with "unacceptable views," terms they now wear proudly. They are convinced their government holds them in contempt— and it's hard to say they are wrong.

Andrew Lawton is the bestselling author of *The Freedom Convoy: The Inside Story of Three Weeks that Shook the World.*

By Justin Ling

"Kanellakos and Brookson were living in different worlds," Paul Wells writes in *An Emergency in Ottawa*.

In early 2022, Steve Kanellakos was Ottawa's city manager and Larry Brookson was responsible for security in the parliamentary precinct. The Freedom Convoy had come to Ottawa and each was trying to deal with it.

Kanellakos had negotiated a plan to move a bunch of upside-down-Canada-flag-waving semi-trailer trucks out of residential neighborhoods and closer to Parliament Hill. Brookson was aghast: he had just finished running through a contingency plan in case one of those trucks was wired to blow the seat of Canadian democracy sky-high.

What is incredible about those three weeks, which Wells summarizes neatly, is how many of those different worlds could fit in Ottawa.

Brookson and Kanellakos lived on neighboring planets: one, trying to bring order and peace to the city's residents; the other, preparing for the worst-case scenario.

On one side of the known universe there were political staffers, eagerly texting each other about the necessary "framing" of the "narrative" of the occupation; on the other end was the kook who conceived the convoy itself, positive his "Memorandum of Understanding" would turf those staffers and let him govern with his pals.

On a cold, noisy moon were residents of downtown apartment buildings debating which patch of their bathroom floor was best insulated from the air horns of the trucks outside; a few hundred light-years away was the well-to-do lawyer who, after arriving on a private jet full of unvaccinated white-collar types, scurried around trying to turn the grassroots occupation into a permanent cash cow.

Implicit in Wells' book and, of course, in the voluminous record of the Public Order Emergency Commission on which it turns, is that getting everyone on the same planet might have alleviated this disaster, maybe averted it altogether.

If the convoy types had understood how miserable life had become for some of those Ottawa residents with disabilities, maybe they would have observed some quiet hours, at least. Or if Prime Minister Justin Trudeau had appreciated how fed up many unvaccinated people felt, maybe, at least, he could have avoided calling them names. Or if Doug Ford had stopped aimlessly drifting through space and decided to govern.

None of that happened. So Canadians, "in some circles," Wells snidely notes, refused to accept that militant anti-vaxxers exist here—they "must be 'Americans.'" (He lets them off too easy: many were convinced it was the Ruskies.) And the convoy participants threw a party, convinced they would be vindicated eventually. And the federal government invoked the *Emergencies Act*, for the first time, because it believed negotiating with the truckers was not an option and saw no other way out.

Wells' lay of the land is succinct, excellent, and a useful exercise, even for those of us familiar with the whole solar system.

He does not, alas, convince me that getting on the same planet would have solved anything. Ottawa police had developed a plan before the *Emergencies Act* was invoked, but it's hard to imagine they could have cleared the convoy as quickly or effectively without it. When the operation finally went down, there were hundreds of officers from across the country who made it possible.

And while there is little to like about the Trudeau government's petulant attitude through much of the crisis, or its attitude towards unvaccinated people broadly, he was right to refuse the invitation to negotiate with the occupiers. The idea that a Hot Tub Debate between himself and some convoy captain, a la Nixon and Krushchev, would have produced anything but frustration and hot air is optimistic, to say the least.

Of course, neither hypothetical can be falsified without travelling through the wormhole. I'll grant that even if the police plan and interaction with the protestors wouldn't have *solved* anything, they may have netted some benefits. And here in our present reality, getting back on the same surface—or, at least, figuring out the particulars of interstellar communication—is a noble and ambitious mission.

I had forgotten, until Wells' pithy reminder, of the brief rebellion by young Quebecois MP Joël Lightbound. He made the alien observation that the government's strategy of wedge, divide, and stigmatize had created the convoy and, worse, was weakening support for the public health apparatus more broadly. That is spectacular backfire. His minders quickly shuffled him away to a topsecret air base outside of Rimouski and returned him to Ottawa in working order, never to speak ill of the government again.

"The hardest thing, when you know how the story ends, is to remember what it felt like not to know how it would end," Wells observes. I can transport myself back there and remember the anger I felt at not just at the unvaccinated but the ones who counseled others to remain, as some at the convoy liked to say, "pureblood." I suppose I'm still angry.

But today's lesson is that anger doesn't need to be an excuse to disconnect. Petty infighting at Ottawa Police headquarters is no excuse to fail the city you serve and which pays your bills. Anger at the people who have acted as irresponsible citizens amidst a deadly pandemic doesn't justify a lack of empathy.

The most unconscionable offenders, however, are the ones who were the subject of this extraordinary review. It may have been cleared, barely, for using the *Emergencies Act*, but the federal government remains insufferably smug about its own role in this imbroglio.

Wells writes: "Stay in Ottawa long enough and you get used to politicians demanding more civility from other people."

Justin Ling is a freelance investigative journalist, author, and writer of the Bug-Eyed and Shameless newsletter.

NOTES

Introduction

1 https://www.wsj.com/articles/covid-origin-china-lab-leak-807b7b0a?mod=e2tw
2 https://www.cnn.com/2023/02/27/politics/covid-origins-doe-assessment-what-matters/index.html
3 https://www.newsweek.com/huge-problem-lab-leak-theory-was-dismissed-conspiracy-ex-who-adviser-1784177
4 https://www.reuters.com/business/healthcare-pharmaceuticals/who-advisors-urge-china-release-all-covid-related-data-after-new-research-2023-03-18/
5 https://www.smithsonianmag.com/smart-news/genetic-evidence-ties-covids-origin-to-raccoon-dogs-180981846/

Chapter One

1 Statista. "Number of coronavirus (COVID-19) cases, recoveries, and deaths worldwide as of June 1, 2021." Statista. Accessed 2021 Jun 1. Available at www.statista.com/statistics/1087466/covid19-cases-recoveries-deaths-worldwide.
2 Apolone G, Montomoli E, Manenti A, Boeri M, et al. "Unexpected detection of SARS-CoV-2 antibodies in the prepandemic period in Italy." Tumori. 2020 Nov 11: 300891620974755.
3 Deslandes A, Berti V, Tandjaoui-Lambotte Y, Chakib Alloui, et al. "SARS-CoV-2 was already spreading in France in late December 2019." Int J Antimicrob Agents. 2020 Jun; 55 (6):106006.
4 https://www.cpha.ca/review-canadas-initial-response-covid-19-pandemic
5 https://www.ourwindsor.ca/news-story/10124148-how-a-toronto-hospital-handled-canada-s-first-covid-19-case-we-didn-t-know-this-was-a-moment-in-history-/

6 https://www.thestar.com/politics/2021/01/24/a-timeline-of-covid-19-in-canada.html

7 https://nationalpost.com/news/politics/canadas-early-covid-19-cases-came-from-the-u-s-not-china-provincial-data-shows

8 https://www.cpha.ca/review-canadas-initial-response-covid-19-pandemic

9 https://www.thestar.com/politics/2021/01/24/a-timeline-of-covid-19-in-canada.html; https://www.cbc.ca/news/health/coronavirus-canada-death-1.5491907

10 https://www.cbc.ca/news/politics/covid19-coronavirus-ottawa-hill-economic-legislation-1.5509178

11 https://www.npr.org/2020/03/28/823292062/who-reviews-available-evidence-on-coronavirus-transmission-through-air

12 https://www.cbc.ca/news/politics/non-medical-masks-covid-19-spread-1.5523321

13 https://www.thestar.com/news/canada/2021/05/07/governments-across-canada-withholding-covid-19-data-to-regulate-public-reaction-to-pandemic-says-access-to-information-advocate.html

14 https://www.bankofcanada.ca/2020/10/staff-analytical-note-2020-22/; https://www.cbc.ca/news/business/covid-economy-changes-1.5618734; https://utpjournals.press/doi/full/10.3138/cpp.2020-072

15 https://www.theglobeandmail.com/canada/article-canadas-medical-workers-scramble-to-find-child-care-amid-covid-1/

16 https://www.cbc.ca/news/canada/north/sourdough-popular-covid-19-1.5529649

17 https://www.thestar.com/politics/federal/2020/05/07/82-of-canadas-covid-19-deaths-have-been-in-long-term-care.html

18 https://www.theguardian.com/world/2020/may/26/canada-care-homes-military-report-coronavirus#:~:text=At%20one%20point%2C%20%E2%80%9Cpatients%20%5B,%2C%20of%20frustration%2C%20of%20grief.

19 https://canoe.com/news/national/long-term-care-cases-made-up-80-of-canadas-covid-19-deaths-in-first-wave

20 https://www.cbc.ca/news/canada/toronto/military-long-term-care-home-report-covid-ontario-1.5585844; https://www.cbc.ca/news/canada/toronto/covid-19-coronavirus-ontario-update-may-26-1.5584665

21 https://canoe.com/news/national/long-term-care-cases-made-up-80-of-canadas-covid-19-deaths-in-first-wave

22 https://www.theglobeandmail.com/canada/article-morning-update-new-federal-long-term-care-standards-wont-be-mandatory/

23 https://torontosun.com/news/local-news/covidiots-trinity-bellwoods-jam-packed-despite-rules

24 https://globalnews.ca/news/7043334/trinity-bellwoods-park-toronto-coronavirus/

25 https://www.yalemedicine.org/news/covid-19-variants-of-concern-omicron
   #:~:text=Alpha%20(B.1.1.7,as%20a%20variant%20of%20concern.

26 https://www.cp24.com/news/ford-reiterates-support-for-lockdown-measures-
   as-ontario-posts-another-record-number-of-covid-19-cases-1.5207188

27 https://www.cbc.ca/news/canada/toronto/covid-19-coronavirus-ontario-
   december-3-icu-numbers-1.5826565

28 https://www.gatesnotes.com/What-you-need-to-know-about-the-COVID-
   19-vaccine

29 https://news.ontario.ca/en/release/59607/ontario-begins-rollout-of-covid-
   19-vaccine

30 https://www.thestar.com/politics/2021/01/24/a-timeline-of-covid-19-in-
   canada.html

31 https://nationalpost.com/news/the-price-of-worship-during-covid-ontario-
   church-is-fined-and-an-alberta-pastor-sits-in-prison

32 https://theconversation.com/covid-19-delta-variant-in-canada-faq-on-
   origins-hotspots-and-vaccine-protection-162653

33 Ibid.

34 https://toronto.ctvnews.ca/ford-warns-ontarians-to-be-very-cautious-after-
   covid-19-third-wave-declared-in-province-1.5348764

35 https://www.nbcnews.com/politics/donald-trump/trump-renews-praise-
   covid-vaccines-one-greatest-achievements-mankind-n1286551

36 https://www.yalemedicine.org/news/covid-19-variants-of-concern-omicron
   #:~:text=Alpha%20(B.1.1.7,as%20a%20variant%20of%20concern.

37 https://globalnews.ca/news/7747134/alberta-government-dissent-covid-19-
   health-rules-caucus-kenney/

38 https://health-infobase.canada.ca/covid-19/vaccination-coverage/

39 https://www.cbc.ca/news/canada/toronto/ontario-covid-vaccine-passport-
   certificate-proof-1.6160728

40 https://www.ontario.ca/page/covid-19-vaccines

41 https://health-infobase.canada.ca/covid-19/vaccine-administration/

42 https://toronto.ctvnews.ca/ontario-reports-first-two-cases-of-omicron-
   covid-19-variant-1.5684897

43 https://twitter.com/CFIB/status/1405197538819465220

44 https://www.nih.gov/news-events/nih-research-matters/bivalent-boosters-
   provide-better-protection-against-severe-covid-19#:~:text=Bivalent%20
   booster%20vaccines%20against%20SARS,previously%20received%20a%20
   different%20booster.

45 https://www.nebraskamed.com/COVID/what-covid-19-variants-are-going-
   around#:~:text=What%20COVID%2D19%20variant%20are,1.1%20and%20
   BQ.1.%22

46 https://www.canada.ca/en/public-health/services/publications/vaccines-
   immunization/national-advisory-committee-immunization-guidance-

additional-covid-19-booster-dose-spring-2023-individuals-high-risk-severe-illness-due-covid-19.html

Chapter Two

1 https://www.bloomberg.com/news/newsletters/2022-06-04/coronavirus-daily-just-how-wildly-are-covid-cases-undercounted

2 https://www.cdc.gov/nchs/pressroom/nchs_press_releases/2022/20220622.htm

3 https://covid19.who.int/

4 https://aircraft.airbus.com/en/aircraft/a320-the-most-successful-aircraft-family-ever/a320ceo#:~:text=With%20a%20versatile%20cabin%20that,of%20up%20to%20180%20travellers.

5 https://www.statista.com/statistics/1362951/super-bowl-attendance/#:~:text=The%202023%20Super%20Bowl%2C%20which,Bowl%20title%20in%20franchise%20history.

6 https://wisevoter.com/state-rankings/states-by-population/

7 Comparing normal rates at which people died to what happened during the pandemic = Provisional death counts and excess mortality, January 2020 to March 2022 https://www150.statcan.gc.ca/n1/daily-quotidien/220609/dq220609e-eng.htm

8 Ibid.

9 Ibid.

10 https://covid19tracker.ca/vaccinationtracker.html

11 https://bmcpublichealth.biomedcentral.com/articles/10.1186/s12889-022-14090-z/tables/1

12 https://www.nytimes.com/2023/02/02/opinion/covid-pandemic-deaths.html

13 https://www.nytimes.com/2023/02/02/opinion/covid-pandemic-deaths.html

14 https://insidemedicine.substack.com/p/data-snapshot-are-we-overcounting

15 https://www.cdc.gov/nchs/nvss/vsrr/covid19/excess_deaths.htm

16 https://www.nytimes.com/2023/02/02/opinion/covid-pandemic-deaths.html

17 https://www.cbc.ca/news/health/covid-testing-shortages-1.5503926#:~:text=A%20key%20to%20slowing%20the,to%20prioritize%20who%20gets%20tested.

18 https://www.mayoclinic.org/diseases-conditions/coronavirus/in-depth/coronavirus-long-term-effects/art-20490351#:~:text=People%20who%20had%20severe%20illness,long%20these%20effects%20might%20last.

19 https://www150.statcan.gc.ca/n1/daily-quotidien/221017/dq221017b-eng.htm

20 https://covidinscotstudy.scot/

21 https://academic.oup.com/jid/advance-article/doi/10.1093/infdis/jiac136/6569364?login=false

22 https://www.cidrap.umn.edu/news-perspective/2022/04/global-data-reveal-half-may-have-long-covid-4-months

23 https://www.thelancet.com/journals/lancet/article/PIIS0140-6736(22)00941-2/fulltext

24 https://www.thelancet.com/journals/eclinm/article/PIIS2589-5370(21)00299-6/fulltext

25 https://www.cdc.gov/coronavirus/2019-ncov/hcp/clinical-care/underlying conditions.html

26 https://www.cdc.gov/coronavirus/2019-ncov/long-term-effects/index.html#:~:text=Some%20people%2C%20especially%20those%20who,kidney%2C%2C%20skin%2C%20and%20brain.

27 https://ccforum.biomedcentral.com/articles/10.1186/s13054-021-03884-z

28 https://www.thoracic.org/about/newsroom/press-releases/resources/lung_abnormalities_after_covid19.pdf

29 https://www.frontiersin.org/articles/10.3389/fimmu.2022.1034159/full

30 https://www.nature.com/articles/d41586-022-02074-3

31 https://press.rsna.org/timssnet/media/pressreleases/14_pr_target.cfm?id=2381

32 https://journals.lww.com/jasn/Fulltext/2021/11000/Kidney_Outcomes_in_Long_COVID.19.aspx

33 Xie, Y. & Al-Aly, Z. Lancet Diabetes Endocrinol. https://doi.org/10.1016/S2213-8587(22)00044-4 (2022)

34 Ibid.

35 London, J.W.; Fazio-Eynullayeva, E.; Palchuk, M.B.; Sankey, P.; McNair, C. Effects of the COVID-19 Pandemic on Cancer-Related Patient Encounters. JCO Clin. Cancer Inform. 2020, 4, 657–665.

36 Richards, M.; Anderson, M. The impact of the COVID-19 pandemic on cancer care. Nat. Cancer 2020, 1, 565–567.

37 Measuring the impact of the COVID-19 pandemic on organized cancer screening and diagnostic follow-up care in Ontario, Canada: A provincial, population-based study. Prev. Med. 2021 Oct;151:106586. doi: 10.1016/j.ypmed.2021.106586.

38 McBain R.K., Cantor J.H. Decline and Rebound in Routine Cancer Screening Rates During the COVID-19 Pandemic. J. Gen. Intern. Med. 2021;36:1829–1831. doi: 10.1007/s11606-021-06660-5.

39 https://www.cma.ca/sites/default/files/pdf/health-advocacy/Deloitte-report-nov2021-EN.pdf

40 Ramsey C.R.F., Karma L.K., Li L., Laura Elizabeth P., Veena S., Scott D. Stage at cancer diagnosis during the COVID-19 pandemic in western Washington state. J. Clin. Oncol. 2021;39:145. doi: 10.1200/JCO.2020.39.28_suppl.145.

41 Sharpless N.E. COVID-19 and cancer. Science. 2020; 368:1290. doi: 10.1126/science.abd3377.

42 https://www.thelancet.com/journals/lanonc/article/PIIS1470-2045(20)30243-6/fulltext
43 Ibid.
44 https://www.cma.ca/sites/default/files/pdf/health-advocacy/Deloitte-report-nov2021-EN.pdf
45 https://www.fraserinstitute.org/sites/default/files/waiting-your-turn-2022.pdf
46 Ibid.

Chapter Three

1 Smetanin et al. (2011). The life and economic impact of major mental illnesses in Canada: 2011-2041. Prepared for the Mental Health Commission of Canada. Toronto: RiskAnalytica
2 https://www.nature.com/articles/s41562-022-01453-0
3 https://www150.statcan.gc.ca/n1/daily-quotidien/220713/dq220713a-eng.htm
4 https://www.ncbi.nlm.nih.gov/pmc/articles/PMC5702385/
5 https://www.who.int/news/item/02-03-2022-covid-19-pandemic-triggers-25-increase-in-prevalence-of-anxiety-and-depression-worldwide
6 https://www.canada.ca/en/public-health/services/publications/diseases-conditions/cycle-2-symptoms-anxiety-depression-covid-19-pandemic.html
7 https://www.sunlife.com/en/newsroom/news-releases/announcement/mental-health-drug-claims-skyrocket-among-young-canadians/123709/#:~:text=Yet%20new%20Sun%20Life%20data,rise%20in%20claims%20at%2013%25.
8 https://www.cma.ca/sites/default/files/pdf/health-advocacy/Deloitte-report-nov2021-EN.pdf
9 Comparison of mental health symptoms before and during the covid-19 pandemic: evidence from a systematic review and meta-analysis of 134 cohorts" by Ying Sun et al.
10 https://www.pollara.com/the-rage-index-looking-at-the-mood-of-canadians/
11 https://theconversation.com/the-governments-use-of-the-emergencies-act-was-found-to-be-reasonable-but-what-are-the-implications-200213
12 https://data-planet.libguides.com/MiseryIndex
13 https://www.statista.com/statistics/1324607/us-misery-index/#:~:text=Due%20to%20high%20levels%20of,high%20rate%20of%2012.6%20percent.
14 https://www.bloomberg.com/news/articles/2022-07-30/midterm-misery-for-biden-as-key-economy-gauge-flags-30-seat-loss
15 https://www.theglobeandmail.com/business/article-misery-index-2022/
16 https://www.kff.org/coronavirus-covid-19/issue-brief/the-implications-of-covid-19-for-mental-health-and-substance-use/

17 https://www.canada.ca/en/health-canada/services/canadian-alcohol-drugs-survey/2019-summary.html
18 https://www.ncbi.nlm.nih.gov/pmc/articles/PMC8200837/
19 https://www.canada.ca/en/public-health/services/publications/healthy-living/infographic-examining-changes-alcohol-cannabis-consumption-stigma-covid-pandemic.html
20 https://www150.statcan.gc.ca/t1/tbl1/en/tv.action?pid=1010001101
21 https://www.thestar.com/news/gta/2022/01/15/doctors-are-noticing-patients-are-drinking-more-fuelling-more-hospitalizations.html
22 https://aasldpubs.onlinelibrary.wiley.com/doi/abs/10.1002/hep.32272
23 https://bmcpsychiatry.biomedcentral.com/articles/10.1186/s12888-022-04185-7
24 https://www.kamloopsthisweek.com/local-news/bc-kamloops-set-grim-record-for-overdose-deaths-in-2021-5045461; https://www.cbc.ca/news/canada/british-columbia/bc-covid-19-weekly-update-february-2-1.6735397
25 https://covid19-sciencetable.ca/sciencebrief/the-impact-of-the-covid-19-pandemic-on-opioid-related-harm-in-ontario/
26 https://www2.gov.bc.ca/assets/gov/birth-adoption-death-marriage-and-divorce/deaths/coroners-service/statistical/illicit-drug.pdf
27 https://www.canada.ca/en/health-canada/services/opioids/data-surveillance-research/modelling-opioid-overdose-deaths-covid-19.html
28 https://www.cdc.gov/drugoverdose/deaths/index.html#:~:text=In%20 2020%2C%2091%2C799%20drug%20overdose,driver%20of%20drug%20 overdose%20deaths.
29 https://www.ama-assn.org/system/files/issue-brief-increases-in-opioid-related-overdose.pdf
30 https://www.apa.org/monitor/2021/03/substance-use-pandemic
31 CMAJ July 11, 2022 194 (26) E919-E920; DOI: https://doi.org/10.1503/cmaj.1096005
32 https://www.ccsa.ca/mental-health-and-substance-use-during-covid-19#:~:text=The%20COVID%2D19%20pandemic%20has,many%20people%20 living%20in%20Canada
33 https://www150.statcan.gc.ca/n1/pub/82-003-x/2022005/article/00002-eng.htm
34 https://www.ccsa.ca/mental-health-and-substance-use-during-covid-19#:~:text=The%20COVID%2D19%20pandemic%20has,many%20 people%20living%20in%20Canada
35 https://www.nature.com/articles/s41562-021-01139-z
36 https://www150.statcan.gc.ca/t1/tbl1/en/tv.action?pid=3510006801& pickMembers%5B0%5D=1.1&cubeTimeFrame.startYear=1990&cube TimeFrame.endYear=2021&referencePeriods=19900101%2C20210101
37 https://www150.statcan.gc.ca/n1/daily-quotidien/221019/dq221019c-eng.htm

38 https://www150.statcan.gc.ca/n1/daily-quotidien/221019/dq221019c-eng.htm
39 https://www150.statcan.gc.ca/n1/daily-quotidien/221019/dq221019c-eng.htm
40 Offord Centre for Child Studies. "Impact of the Covid-19 pandemic on Ontario families with children: Findings from the initial lockdown." McMaster University. 2020 Sept. Available at https://assets.documentcloud.org/documents/7203244/OPS-Executive-Report-v6-FINAL.pdf.
41 https://thehub.ca/2023-02-16/its-not-just-toronto-violent-crime-is-a-national-problem/
42 https://news.gov.bc.ca/files/Prolific_Offender_Report_BCFNJC_submission.pdf
43 https://globalnews.ca/news/9505043/ttc-crime-toronto-december/#:~:text=The%20figures%20mean%20that%2C%20on,1.85%20every%20million%20in%20November.
44 https://toronto.ctvnews.ca/terrible-tragedy-politicians-speak-out-following-fatal-stabbing-of-teen-at-toronto-subway-station-1.6330685
45 Ibid. p. 43
46 https://www.canada.ca/en/public-health/services/diseases/coronavirus-disease-covid-19/vaccines
47 https://health-infobase.canada.ca/covid-19/vaccine-administration/#a5
48 https://health-infobase.canada.ca/covid-19/vaccine-safety/summary.html
49 https://health-infobase.canada.ca/covid-19/vaccine-safety/#seriousNon Serious
50 https://www.ema.europa.eu/en/news/astrazenecas-covid-19-vaccine-ema-finds-possible-link-very-rare-cases-unusual-blood-clots-low-blood
51 https://health-infobase.canada.ca/covid-19/vaccine-administration/#a2
52 Ibid.
53 Ibid.
54 https://jamanetwork.com/journals/jama/fullarticle/2801828
55 https://cca-reports.ca/wp-content/uploads/2023/01/Report-Fault-Lines-digital.pdf

Chapter Four

1 https://www.nimh.nih.gov/health/topics/post-traumatic-stress-disorder-ptsd
2 https://www.ncbi.nlm.nih.gov/pmc/articles/PMC7227560/
3 https://pubmed.ncbi.nlm.nih.gov/33910674/
4 "Multi-organ impairment and Long COVID: a 1-year prospective, longitudinal cohort study" by Andrea Dennis, et al. 14 February 2023, Journal of the Royal Society of Medicine. DOI: 10.1177/01410768231154703
5 https://toronto.ctvnews.ca/nearly-1-in-2-nurses-in-ontario-considering-

leaving-their-jobs-poll-1.6013201; https://rnao.ca/news/media-releases/
results-of-nursing-survey-point-to-an-alarming-exodus-from-the-profession

6 https://angusreid.org/canada-health-care-family-doctors-shortage/
7 https://www.ox.ac.uk/news/2023-01-31-covid-19-leading-cause-death-children-and-young-people-us
8 https://www.gstic.org/expert-story/how-covid-19-has-exposed-the-challenges-for-technology-in-education/
9 https://www.unicef.org/press-releases/two-thirds-worlds-school-age-children-have-no-Internet-access-home-new-unicef-itu
10 https://www.nature.com/articles/s41562-022-01506-4
11 https://www.nytimes.com/2023/01/30/health/covid-education-children.html
12 https://www.cmaj.ca/content/194/26/E919
13 https://www.who.int/news-room/fact-sheets/detail/adolescent-mental-health
14 Ibid.
15 Reginald D. Williams II et al., The Impact of COVID-19 on Older Adults: Findings from the 2021 International Health Policy Survey of Older Adults (Commonwealth Fund, Sept. 2021). https://doi.org/10.26099/mqsp-1695; https://www.commonwealthfund.org/publications/surveys/2021/sep/impact-covid-19-older-adults
16 ibid.
17 https://www.mckinsey.com/capabilities/people-and-organizational-performance/our-insights/a-military-veteran-knows-why-your-employees-are-leaving
18 https://www.pewresearch.org/social-trends/2022/02/16/covid-19-pandemic-continues-to-reshape-work-in-america/
19 https://www.ctvnews.ca/lifestyle/canadians-told-us-why-they-changed-jobs-during-covid-here-s-how-their-lives-have-changed-since-1.6243731
20 https://tech.co/news/tim-cook-apple-return-office-mandate
21 https://www.bnnbloomberg.ca/canadian-employers-face-resistance-as-they-seek-to-increase-office-days-1.1881692
22 https://www.mckinsey.com/featured-insights/future-of-work/the-future-of-work-after-covid-19
23 https://www.macrotrends.net/countries/NAC/north-america/unemployment-rate
24 Tom Bundervoet et al. "The Short-Term Impacts of COVID-19 on Households in Developing Countries: An Overview Based on a Harmonized Data Set of High-Frequency Surveys," Policy Research Working Paper 9582, World Bank, Washington, DC, 2021; Markus P. Goldstein, et al. "The Global State of Small Business during COVID-19: Gender Inequalities," Let's Talk Development (blog), September 8, 2020.
25 https://www.oecd.org/economic-outlook/november-2022/

26 https://www.fao.org/3/al936e/al936e00.pdf

27 https://www150.statcan.gc.ca/n1/daily-quotidien/230117/dq230117b-eng.htm

28 chrome-extension://efaidnbmnnnibpcajpcglclefindmkaj/https://cdn.dal.ca/content/dam/dalhousie/pdf/sites/agri-food/Canada%27s%20Food%20Price%20Report%202023_Digital.pdf

29 https://www.theglobeandmail.com/business/article-canada-office-vacancy-rate/

Chapter Five

1 The Commonwealth Fund Report: US Health Care from a Global Perspective, 2022: Accelerating Spending, Worsening OutcomesJanuary 2023. https://www.commonwealthfund.org/publications/issue-briefs/2023/jan/us-health-care-global-perspective-2022.

2 The Commonwealth Fund Report: Mirror, Mirror 2021: Reflecting Poorly, 2021.https://www.commonwealthfund.org/publications/fund-reports/2021/aug/mirror-mirror-2021-reflecting-poorly

3 https://nccdh.ca/images/uploads/comments/Economic_Arguments_EN_April_28.pdf

4 https://www.tfah.org/report-details/publichealthfunding2020/

5 https://www.canada.ca/en/institutes-health-research/news/2022/01/government-of-canada-makes-significant-investment-in-research-to-transform-public-health-for-canadians.html

6 https://www.fda.gov/drugs/special-features/why-you-need-take-your-medications-prescribed-or-instructed